ECOBEAUTY

ECOBEAUTY

Scrubs, Rubs, Masks, and Bath Bombs for You and Your Friends

by Lauren Cox with Janice Cox

Photography by Angie Cao

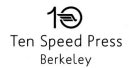

Ten Speed Press
Berkeley

To our family who is always there for us.
You all make a difference in our world!

Copyright © 2009 by Lauren Cox and Janice Cox
Photographs copyright © 2009 by Angie Cao

All rights reserved.
Published in the United States by Ten Speed Press, an imprint of the Crown Publishing Group,
a division of Random House, Inc., New York.
www.crownpublishing.com
www.tenspeed.com

Ten Speed Press and the Ten Speed Press colophon are registered trademarks of Random House, Inc.

Library of Congress Cataloging-in-Publication Data

Cox, Lauren.
  Ecobeauty : scrubs, rubs, masks, and bath bombs for you and your friends / by Lauren Cox with Janice Cox.
      p. cm.
  Includes bibliographical references and index.
  Summary: "100 fresh and eco-friendly projects for body, face, and hair, from up-and-coming natural beauty expert, teenager Lauren Cox and her mother, leading home beauty author Janice Cox"
—Provided by publisher.
  1. Beauty, Personal. 2. Herbal cosmetics. I. Cox, Janice. II. Title.
  RA776.98.C69 2009
  646.7'2--dc22

                      2009005578

ISBN 978-1-58008-852-7

Printed in China, text printed on recycled paper (100% PCW with soy-based inks)

Design by Chloe Rawlins
Prop styling by Daniele Kent Maxwell

10 9 8 7 6 5 4 3 2 1

First Edition

Contents

For the Hair 107

Gift Giving 125

Make a Difference! ❋ 148
Index ❋ 149

Acknowledgments

We were very lucky to have so many amazing people be a part of this book.

Thanks to all of our friends and family members who helped us test the recipes and gave us their feedback and opinions, especially Marie and Ray Cox, who always support us in everything we do.

Thanks to our agent, Laurie Harper, whose enthusiasm and support is never-ending.

To our editor, Lisa Westmoreland, who shared our vision and passion for *EcoBeauty* from the start, thank you for everything.

A special thank-you to Chloe Rawlins for your cover and interior design, Angie Cao for your photography, Daniele Kent Maxwell for your help in styling all our shots, and Jasmine Star for your eagle-eyed copyediting.

And a big thanks to everyone at Ten Speed Press for your time and effort; writing a book is definitely a team effort, and we had the best team ever. You are all naturally beautiful!

—Lauren and Janice

Introduction

Creating your own scrubs, rubs, masks, bath bombs, and other body care products is fun, easy, and cost-effective. Plus, homemade, natural beauty products will make your skin and hair look amazing. They also make great gifts for family and friends. I loved putting together this collection of recipes. Many of them are things I use every day, and all of the ingredients are easy to find. You may have to go to a natural food store for some of them, like essential oils and natural clay, but the majority of the recipes call for common kitchen items such as milk, honey, salt, sugar, baking soda, tea, and vinegar.

I grew up using homemade beauty products because my mom is Janice Cox, a writer and expert on natural beauty, and my sister, Marie, and I were her recipe testers. I always had homemade lip balms in my backpack and spa-themed birthday parties. One year my mom even put a Barbie doll on my cake—floating in a fluffy frosting bubble bath and with cucumber slices over her eyes! You may also have used homemade treatments that your mother taught you, such as using a baking soda rinse on your hair or treating a sunburn with aloe—or maybe not, and this is a whole new world for you to discover.

Today I'm a freshman in college, but I still find time to put together home beauty treatments. When my skin looks a bit dull, I mix up a quick scrub of yogurt and cornmeal, or if I'm stressed-out after a long day of tests, I dab on some scented oil, listen to my iPod, and relax. I've even gotten my roommates into the habit of home facials, manicures, and hair rinses.

I'm also on a pretty tight budget, and making your own products and treatments definitely saves money. Some girls spend $20 per week on salon manicures and pedicures. Learning to do your own could save you over a thousand dollars a year! And for mere pennies, you can make products that would cost dollars in a store. Plus, you have the benefit of not having to wait for an appointment or drive to a salon.

Making some of these recipes is also a fun and relaxing way to spend time with friends. I've gotten together with my sports teams, roommates, and best girlfriends for spa parties and gift-making sessions, which is an especially great idea around the holidays. You can create Halloween facial masks, holiday bath salts, or birthday bath bombs. They make truly unique gifts, and your friends and family will be impressed that you made them yourself.

Making your own body care products will also make you a smarter shopper. You'll start reading labels and looking at the list of ingredients. Sometimes I just do this for fun, and other times I'm trying to figure out how to make my favorite product at home. I don't like a long list of ingredients. In fact, the shorter the list, the better for your skin and hair (and the planet!). Also, the ingredients are usually listed by amount, from most to least. Sometimes chemical names are used on commercial products, but a chemical name isn't necessarily a bad thing. For example, sodium chloride is table salt, bicarbonate of soda is baking soda, and tocopherol is vitamin E. You can easily find websites and books that are good resources on cosmetic ingredients. Use them to check out the ingredients in the products you use; you might be surprised at what you're putting on your skin and hair.

These days, being green is cool. I don't drive a hybrid car or live in a solar-powered dorm, but I do reuse plastic and glass containers to package the products I make. Creating your own cosmetics also means less waste. If you've ever opened up a store-bought product you know what I mean. They're usually in a plastic container inside a cardboard box that's wrapped in plastic. Plus, using all-natural ingredients means fewer harmful chemicals going into our landfills or down our drains and into our water supply. So even small lifestyle changes like using natural ingredients with less packaging can help make the world a better place.

I hope you enjoy using this book. I'm excited for you to get started, but I must warn you: Home beauty is a bit addictive, and you won't look at food the same way. These days it's hard for me to throw out any leftover morning oatmeal, as it makes a great facial mask, or to shop for tea without thinking of it as a toner. *EcoBeauty* offers many great ways to look and feel your best while also making a difference in the world, so let's get started!

BE A LABEL READER

Here are some tips when looking for truly natural products to use on your skin and hair:

✳ Just because the label says "natural" doesn't mean the product is either natural or high-quality. There are currently no laws that require companies to have all natural ingredients in their products to label them natural.

✳ The FDA requires companies to use Latin and scientific names for their ingredients, so even if you don't recognize the names or can't pronounce them, it doesn't mean they aren't natural.

✳ Using one or several natural ingredients does not make a product natural or high-quality. Look for products with smaller lists of ingredients and names you recognize.

✳ Be careful if you see warning labels or cautions on your cosmetic products. This is usually a giveaway that the product isn't natural.

Home Beauty Basics

The recipes in this book are easy to make. If you enjoy cooking and crafts, you'll be able to master all of them. Making your own beauty treatments is a lot like following a recipe in a cookbook. Make sure you have all of the ingredients and materials ahead of time. You don't want to get started only to discover that you don't have something you need. Also, because these recipes are for products and treatments you're going to use on your skin and hair, I suggest that you do a spot test first, especially if you have a known food allergy. If you're allergic to tomatoes, chances are using them in a face mask recipe could also cause a reaction. If you're super sensitive, it may even be a good idea to check with your doctor before using a new product or ingredient.

All of the ingredients called for in this book are common and should be easy to find. Many of them are foods that you can buy in most grocery stores. I used standard cooking measures and equipment, including a microwave, blender, and pots and pans, to make all of the recipes in this book.

Shopping for ingredients is fun, especially because of the surprising things you sometimes find along the way. I buy the majority of my ingredients at my local grocery store, but I also like to shop at Asian markets, natural food stores, farmers' markets, and import shops.

MY TEN GO-TO HOME BEAUTY TREATMENTS

This is my top ten list of homemade beauty treatments and ideas that I can't live without!

1. **Sugar scrub:** When I want a bit more scrubbing power, I add a teaspoon of granulated sugar to my favorite cleanser before washing my face.

2. **Honey hair mask:** Pure honey does wonders to restore moisture to dry hair.

3. **Bath salts:** If I'm stressed-out, a relaxing soak always puts me at ease.

4. **Nail oil:** Soaking my nails in olive oil makes them strong and flexible.

5. **Green tea toner:** I use green tea to keep my complexion clean and clear and help combat breakouts.

6. **Lip balm:** Natural lip balms made from cocoa butter and coconut oil help keep my lips soft and smooth.

7. **Baking soda:** Baking soda is an inexpensive ingredient that works wonders on everything from treating smelly feet to deeply cleansing hair.

8. **White vinegar:** If you really want to get rid of rough skin on your feet and soften them, soaking them in a basin of warm water with a cup of white vinegar will do the trick.

9. **Clay masks:** To really clean my face and pores, I love a fresh, homemade clay mask.

10. **Body scrubs:** Once a week I use a good body scrub to keep my skin fresh and clear. An easy mixture is equal parts of light oil and kosher salt. A loofah also works well.

Ingredients

There are so many wonderful ingredients out there that I won't try to list them all in this section. Instead, I'll list those I consider to be beauty staples—things you should always have on hand.

ALOE VERA GEL This soothing natural gel from the aloe vera plant is one of the oldest skin care ingredients and has been used since ancient times to treat and heal the skin. It can be added to lotions, creams, and lip balms. The sap is about 99 percent water; the remaining 1 percent contains many compounds that promote healing, including vitamins, amino acids, and enzymes. Aloe has been found to improve the way our skin hydrates itself. It is also naturally soothing and can be massaged into sunburned skin for a cooling treatment. Many people keep a small aloe plant in their homes to treat minor cuts and scrapes, because of its antibacterial and anti-inflammatory properties. You can simply snip off a leaf and split it open to expose the cool, clear gel.

AVOCADOS Avocados are rich in natural oils, protein, and vitamins, so they make a great facial mask for very dry skin. They can also be used as a hair mask to rehydrate dry tresses. Always save the avocado pit; it makes a good massage tool, or you can grind it up to add to body scrub recipes for extra exfoliating power. First chop the pit into pieces, then process it in a coffee grinder or food processor until it has a texture similar to cornmeal.

BAKING SODA Baking soda is a pantry staple that also has many uses in body care. It can be used as a tooth powder, hair rinse, deodorant, and bath additive. It's also an old-fashioned treatment for sunburn and insect bites. As a cleansing hair rinse it can't be beat; it really helps dissolve any residue left on your hair from styling gels or sprays and gets it squeaky clean.

TIPS FOR LOOKING AND FEELING YOUR BEST EVERY DAY

* Get plenty of sleep. Too many all-night study sessions will show.

* Exercise regularly: walk, run, bike, or dance—whatever it takes to get you moving and help you stay fit.

* Eat right. Fast food is cheap and easy, but there are so many fresh and healthy choices.

* Drink plenty of water and water-based drinks. Skip the soda.

* Keep your skin and hair clean and well hydrated.

* Protect your body from the sun by using a good sunscreen daily.

* Brush and floss your teeth twice a day.

* Exfoliate your body weekly to keep your skin fresh and healthy.

* Take good care of your hands and feet.

* Smile!

BEESWAX Beeswax, which bees produce to make their honeycombs, is the base for many creams, lotions, and lip balms. It's highly regarded as a cosmetics ingredient because of its germ-killing properties, and because it forms a protective barrier on the skin that really locks in moisture. It's usually available wherever fresh honey is sold; try your local natural food store or farmers' market.

CASTOR OIL Castor oil, made from the seed of the castor oil plant, is a pale unscented oil that is excellent for use on your hair, nails, and lips. It is one of the few oils that mixes easily with alcohol, so it is often used in cologne and perfume recipes. It can be found in the health care section of the grocery store and at most drugstores.

COCOA BUTTER I like cocoa butter because it smells like chocolate, and in fact, it is a key ingredient in chocolate. It's also a super skin softener, so it's frequently used in bath products, skin scrubs, lip balms, and body lotions. Cocoa butter also helps diminish scars and stretch marks. When using cocoa butter in recipes, it is useful to chop it up into small pieces or grate it using a kitchen grater so that it is easier to work with and measure.

CORNSTARCH Cornstarch is a fine, white powder made from corn. It can be used as a body powder, in facial masks, and as a thickener when making gels and lotions.

ESSENTIAL OILS Essential oils, which are often associated with the practice of aromatherapy, come in a variety of scents and blends. Although they're a bit expensive, they're highly concentrated, so you only need a drop or two in most recipes. I like to keep small bottles of lavender and peppermint oil in my purse. I use the lavender scent to relax and calm my mind and body and the peppermint scent for an instant energizer.

EXTRACTS Flavored extracts differ from flavored and scented oils because they are alcohol based. Their scent does not last as long as that of oils, but they are useful when you want a lighter, non-greasy mixture without added oil, and they often cost less than scented or flavored oils. They can be found in the baking section of your grocery store. I like to use pure vanilla extract just by itself as a light evening scent. Just dab a few drops behind your ears and people will want to know what you're wearing!

HONEY Honey is another ingredient that's useful from head to toe. It can be used as a hair conditioner, as a skin treatment, and in the bath. Honey is a humectant, meaning it holds moisture, so it's useful for rehydrating dry skin and hair. It also has antibacterial properties, so it's impossible for bacteria to survive in it.

LEMONS I love the fresh, clean scent of lemons. They contain citric acid, which can keep your skin healthy by killing bacteria. It also helps soften typical rough skin problem spots, such as elbows, knees, and feet. Fresh lemon juice can be used to highlight your hair naturally in the sun; just be careful not to overdo, as it can dry your hair out. As with many ingredients, fresh is best—but you can also use frozen or bottled lemon juice.

LIQUID SOAP Any soap can be made into liquid soap by simply dissolving it in water. I suggest using equal parts grated soap and water. For a thicker mixture use more soap, and for a thinner one, more water. You may also add a tablespoon of vegetable glycerin for every cup of liquid soap, which will act as a humectant, keeping the soap saturated with the water. You can also purchase liquid soaps; just look for brands that are all natural and have the fewest number of ingredients. I like to use castile-style soap, which is usually made with natural oils such as olive and almond.

MILK Dairy products such as sour cream, yogurt, and milk are all classic skin cleansers and softeners. The lactic acid in dairy products helps clear away surface debris, and the fats and proteins soothe dry skin. Always use whole-milk dairy products, and be sure to rinse your skin well after using dairy products so that you don't smell like spoiled milk! You can also substitute soy, almond, goat, or hemp milk in many of the recipes that call for cow's milk.

NATURAL OILS I love using natural oils to treat my skin and hair, and there are so many available at grocery stores that it can be hard to choose. I use them all, from almond to walnut. You can use basic oils like sunflower, canola, and olive oil, but it's also fun to experiment with new and exotic oils, such as macadamia, coconut, palm, and apricot kernel oil. I'm sure you'll discover your own favorites. Light oils such as almond, sunflower, and canola can be used as face, hair, and all-over-body oils. Heavier oils such as coconut, dark sesame, and palm should be used in body butters and lip balms and for treating rough skin spots such as feet and elbows. Some oils, such as olive and sesame, come in both light and heavy varieties.

ROLLED OATS Oatmeal is amazing for soothing and softening the skin. In fact, you may remember that an old summer camp cure for poison oak was an oatmeal bath. It's especially good for sensitive skin; many people who can't use soap can use oatmeal in its place. Look for inexpensive rolled oats or steel-cut oats in the cereal aisle.

SALT Salt is a good disinfectant and skin scrub. Salt rubs and scrubs are popular spa treatments and work really well for getting your skin super clean. Soaking in the tub with bath salts is relaxing and also good for sore muscles. I don't recommend using salt on your face, as it's too harsh and drying.

SUGAR Sugar scrubs are becoming as popular as salt scrubs for cleansing and exfoliating. Mixed together with a light cleanser or natural oil, sugar works really well at getting your skin clean and isn't drying like salt can be. I like to use raw sugar when making scrubs, but granulated and brown sugar also work well.

TEA Tea is another multipurpose ingredient. Like baking soda and honey, it can be used all over your body. There are so many types to choose from, and they all work well as hair rinses and skin toners, in baths, and as additions to creams and lotions. I personally love using green and white tea.

VITAMIN E OIL Vitamin E, or tocopherol, can be found in many vegetable oils. Vitamin E oil can be used alone as a moisturizer, and since it is very thick and sticky, it is best used on small areas. It is also believed to help fade scars. Vitamin E oil is also a natural preservative for your homemade beauty products, and can be purchased at most drugstores and grocery stores. If you can't find the oil in bottles, you can purchase the vitamin capsules and prick them with a pin to release the oil if you only need a small amount.

WATER Water is the most common of all beauty ingredients. You can't beat a splash of cool water to refresh your skin or a good soak in the tub to relax your body. One of the best beauty tips of all is to keep your skin and hair hydrated from the inside by drinking plenty of pure water. Remember to use pure or filtered water when making homemade beauty products, as you don't want to introduce any foreign ingredients or bacteria into your recipes. If you have any doubts about your water quality, you can boil it first and let it cool completely, or use distilled water.

WITCH HAZEL Witch hazel is a classic old-fashioned astringent that my grandmother still uses. It's easy to find in the skin care section of your grocery store or drugstore and can be used in creating astringents, toners, after-bath splashes, and colognes.

ECO TIP: It's easy to find cute containers for all of your natural cosmetic products—just look in your recycling bin. Clean your empty bottles and jars with lots of dish detergent and a good scrubbing. You can spruce them up by painting jar lids or buying new corks and stoppers for bottles at your local hardware store. Print up cute labels on your computer or write them on scraps of recycled paper and apply them to your containers with a bit of glue or string. You can also decorate your containers by gluing on small stones, seashells, or photos. Have fun and be creative!

Equipment

As mentioned, I use common kitchen tools and equipment for making my beauty treatments. Here's a list of the basics you should have on hand for the recipes in this book:

* Sharp knives

* Measuring cups and spoons

* Glass ovenproof measuring cups with pouring spouts

* Mixing bowls

* Funnels

* Fine-mesh sieve

* Grater

* Steel or enamel pots

* Old muffin or mini loaf pans

* Blender or food processor

* Coffee grinder

* Microwave

* Stove or heating element

* Assorted bottles, jars, spray bottles, and other containers for packaging

Basic Storage Guidelines

Homemade beauty products call for the same basic care and storage guidelines as commercial body care products, with the exception of recipes or treatments that contain fresh foods. Those should always be refrigerated between uses and usually don't have a long shelf life. Here are some simple tips:

* Store your products in clean containers.

* Keep your fingers out of the products. Pour or spoon the mixture out of the container to avoid introducing germs and bacteria.

* Store your products in a cool, dry, dark place. Heat and light can shorten their shelf life, so don't keep them on your windowsill!

* Leftover products that contain fresh foods should be stored in the refrigerator. Discard them if you think they've spoiled.

* If the product separates, no problem. You can usually just give it a quick stir to mix it up again.

SAFETY

Use caution when handling hot oils and waxes, as they can burn your skin. When using products in the bathroom, you may want to lay a towel on the floor for easier cleanup. When using oil-rich products in the tub or shower, be extra careful not to slip and fall.

Although most of these recipes contain some edible ingredients, some also contain essential oils and other ingredients that aren't edible and could make you ill if ingested. Use caution and avoid applying facial masks and scrubs too close to your mouth. If you do experience a reaction to a certain recipe, ingredient, or product, check with your doctor.

* If something smells or looks bad, it probably is. It's better to throw it out and make a new batch than to spread it on your skin.

* It's hard to predict how long a product will last, as it depends on how it's handled, but most of the recipes in this book will last until you use them up. Dry products last the longest because it's harder for bacteria to grow in a dry environment.

Shopping

Shopping for ingredients is one of my favorite hobbies. I think it's because I grew up shopping for body care products and ingredients with my mom. I love new products and packaging ideas and always enjoy discovering new ingredients. I remember that when we went on family vacations, we always had to hit the local grocery stores. We've brought back tomato soap and cactus shampoo from Mexico, kukui nut oil from Hawaii, spices from Egypt, and honey lip balm from Germany. Here are a few of my favorite places to find ingredients at home.

GROCERY STORES You'll find the majority of the ingredients featured in this book in your local grocery store. I'm lucky as my store also has a natural food section, so I can find all of the basics as well as some fun organic ingredients all in one place. Look in the skin care section for Epsom salts, witch hazel, and cocoa butter.

NATURAL FOOD STORES Natural food stores also have a good selection and often sell things in bulk. They're a good source for natural clays, essential oils, hemp products, and henna. They're also a good place to shop for natural beauty products or to get ideas for gift giving.

DRUGSTORES For skin care basics and beauty tools such as loofahs, manicure gear, cotton balls, and bath brushes, you can't beat your neighborhood drugstore.

ETHNIC MARKETS Asian, Mexican, and Indian markets are all good and cheap sources of exotic ingredients. From floral waters and seaweed to spices and natural oils, it's fun to discover what these shops sell. I've also found interesting beauty products that make great additions to gift baskets, such as donkey milk soap, jasmine water, and gunpowder green tea.

FARMERS' MARKETS For fresh, local, and in-season produce, your local farmers' market is a great place to shop. Not only will you find fruits and vegetables that you may not see at your local grocery store, such as sugar pumpkins, quince, or green tomatoes, it's also a handy spot to pick up beeswax and fresh herbs.

DOLLAR STORES The dollar store is my latest obsession. You can find so many fun, cheap containers and baskets that are perfect for presenting your unique homemade gifts. You can also find towels, washcloths, sponges, and other fun bath supplies, as well as small containers, ice cube trays, and Popsicle molds you can use to shape your soaps and bath bombs. Plus, how can you go wrong for a dollar?

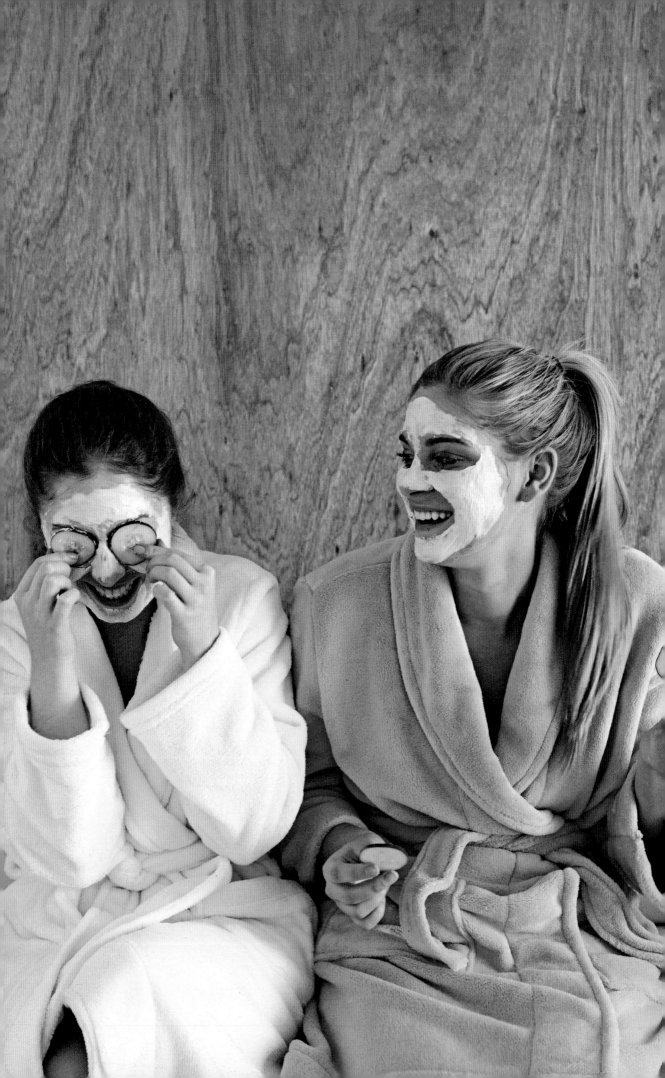

FOR THE FACE

Your face and your complexion are an important part of your identity and how you feel about yourself. It's the one part of your body you can't conceal—unless you want to run around in a ski mask or last year's Halloween disguise, which would not be very cool. Fortunately, clean, healthy skin is easy to achieve and maintain. I know what it's like to wake up with a sudden facial eruption or to live for weeks behind a layer of makeup, hoping no one will notice your skin. But I've also learned that with a little bit of complexion TLC and the right diet you can face the world with confidence!

First of all, it's important to understand what type of skin you have: normal, oily, or dry. However, most of us don't fall neatly into one category or another but instead have a combination of skin types. In fact, your skin type can change with weather, sports activities, and even stress. Here's a simple way to discover your skin type. Before cleansing your skin, blot the oiliest part with a clean white tissue, then examine the tissue. If you can really notice the oil on the tissue, then you have oily skin; if there's just a small amount of oil, you have normal skin; and if there's no oil at all, your skin is dry. Many teens have combination skin, where the forehead and nose area (known as the T-zone) are oily and the cheeks are normal or dry. Understanding your skin type is important, as it will help you choose recipes and products to care for it.

The skin care basics of keeping it clean, full of moisture, and protected from the sun are especially important for your face, but the products you use are a matter of personal choice. At a minimum, you need to use a good cleanser, moisturizer, and sun protection daily. You'll want to use a mild facial scrub and mask weekly. You may also want to use a toner or astringent daily as an extra cleansing step or as a quick way to freshen up during the day.

Keeping your skin clean is important, as this allows it to function more efficiently and look healthier. What you use to cleanse your face is a matter of personal choice. Simple soap and water works for me, but you may choose to use alternatives to soap, like oatmeal or plain yogurt. And your mom is right; you should never go to bed with a dirty face! You need to remove all of the dirt and debris from the day and let your skin breathe and rest at night. There really is such a thing as "beauty sleep."

Toners and astringents are a great addition to your skin care regime. They help deeply cleanse the skin and remove any traces of other cleansers. They also help restore the skin's natural pH, or acidity, which is important for combating surface bacteria and keeping your complexion clear. Astringents are usually alcohol based, making them a bit harsher on the skin and more suited to oily skin types. Toners and fresheners are water based and more appropriate for normal and dry skin types; they can also be used throughout the day to energize and clean your skin.

One word you will hear a lot when it comes to skin care is *exfoliation*. This is a

BEAUTY SMARTS: WHAT DOES SPF MEAN? SPF stands for sun protection factor, and the SPF number tells you how much sun protection the product will provide. For example, if your skin usually turns pink in 10 minutes out in the sun, an SPF of 8 will give you 8 times the protection, so you can be in the sun for 80 minutes. Likewise, an SPF of 15 would give you 150 minutes of protection. Remember, it's always a good idea to be protected. The sun is your skin's greatest enemy!

step that many people don't do or don't do regularly. Exfoliation involves gently scrubbing your skin and removing the oldest dead skin cells. Exfoliating your skin weekly will help unclog your pores and keep your skin really clean. There are several simple scrubs you can use that work well for all skin types, such as superfine sugar, cornmeal, ground nuts, and wheat germ. People with oily or normal skin can use scrubs weekly; those with dry or sensitive skin may want to exfoliate their skin once every two weeks.

Facial masks are another fun and effective weekly beauty treatment that will keep your skin clean and glowing. There are many different types of masks, and the advantage of making your own is that you can create a mask suited to your skin's needs. For example, if you're stressed-out and your skin is reflecting that, you'll want to choose a calming and cleansing mask, like one made with fresh strawberries. But if your skin is really dry or maybe sunburned, you should use soothing and moisturizing ingredients, like aloe or avocado.

I cannot overstress the importance of sun protection. Skin cancer is on the rise among young women, yet it's preventable if you take the right precautions. Use a good sunscreen on your face every day; even during wintertime and cloudy days the sun is still out. A good sunscreen is something you'll have to purchase because they're hard to make at home using household ingredients. Look for products that help block both UVA and UVB rays, and look for these three ingredients in particular: titanium dioxide, zinc oxide, or avobenzene. According to the FDA, these are the only ingredients that give full-spectrum protection to your skin.

TEN TIPS FOR AN AWESOME COMPLEXION

Here are ten simple things you can do for a clean, clear, healthy face:

1. Eat a balanced diet full of fiber, fruits, and vegetables.

2. Keep your hands off of your face and keep your cell phone and headphones clean.

3. Drink plenty of clear liquids and water and avoid drinking too much soda, which is full of sodium, and usually caffeine, sugar, and artificial ingredients.

4. Always protect your skin from the sun!

5. Never go to bed with a dirty face. Always remove all makeup and wash your face with a mild cleanser before bed. Especially after a night out, your skin will thank you in the morning.

6. Always get your "beauty sleep"; lack of sleep can add to stress and cause breakouts.

7. Never squeeze or pop a pimple.

8. Use a facial mask appropriate for your skin type weekly.

9. Gently exfoliate dead skin and surface debris weekly or biweekly, depending on your skin type.

10. When it comes to makeup, less is definitely more. And again, your skin will thank you.

Oh Soy! Cleanser

Soybeans are rich in isoflavones, which are natural plant compounds that act like the female hormone estrogen. They're thought to slow down the aging of the skin, explaining why soy has become such a popular skin care ingredient. This soothing and calming cleanser is perfect for those with sensitive skin. And because the honey helps kill any bacteria, it's also great for people with troubled or acne-prone skin.

1 cup soy milk
1/2 cup rolled oats
1 tablespoon honey

Put all of the ingredients in a blender and blend on high speed until smooth and creamy. Pour the cleanser into a clean jar with a tight-fitting lid. Store this cleanser in the refrigerator between uses. It will keep for 2 to 3 weeks.

To use, place a small amount in the palm of your hand, then gently massage it into your skin. Rinse well with warm water, then pat your skin dry.

Yield: 8 ounces

Honey Bear Cleanser

Honey is a skin superstar. It's a humectant, meaning that it attracts moisture and helps your skin retain moisture. Plus, it helps to control breakouts because of its antibacterial properties. I love to buy honey in the cute plastic bears; when I use up all the honey, I reuse the containers for my homemade honey beauty products and simply glue a label on the front and tie a bow around the top.

1/4 cup honey
1/4 cup water
2 tablespoons liquid soap

Gently stir all of the ingredients together, being careful not to beat the mixture, as this will cause it to foam up. Pour the cleanser into a clean plastic honey bear container or a container with a pour spout or pump.

To use, pour a small amount in the palm of your hand, then massage it gently into your skin or even your hair. Rinse thoroughly with warm water, then pat dry.

Yield: 5 ounces

QUICK TIP: If you have a breakout, dab a bit of honey on the irritated spots after washing your face and before going to bed. You'll notice a difference in the morning.

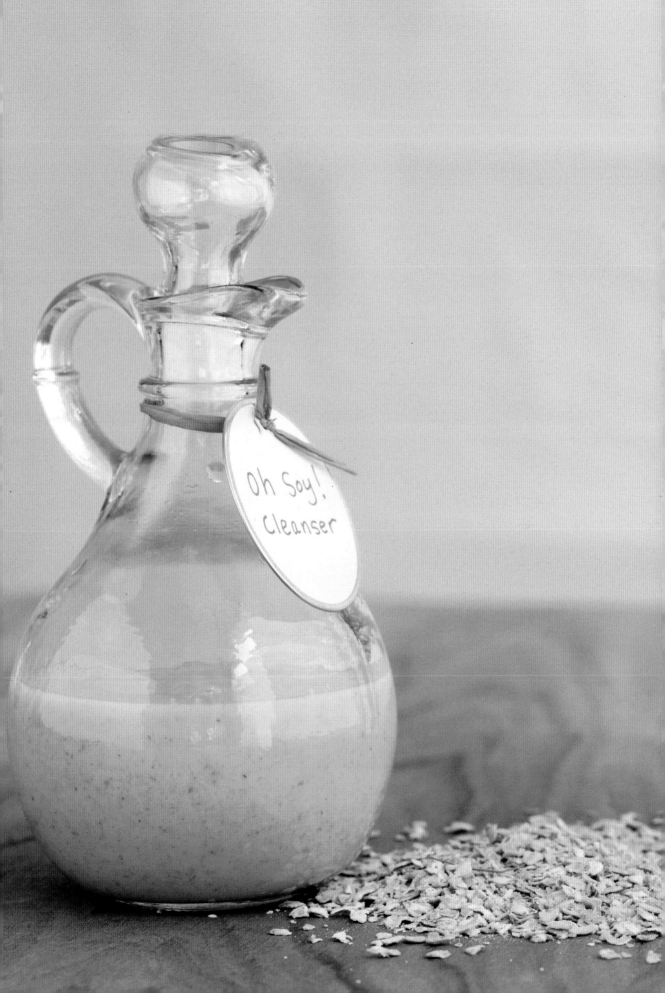

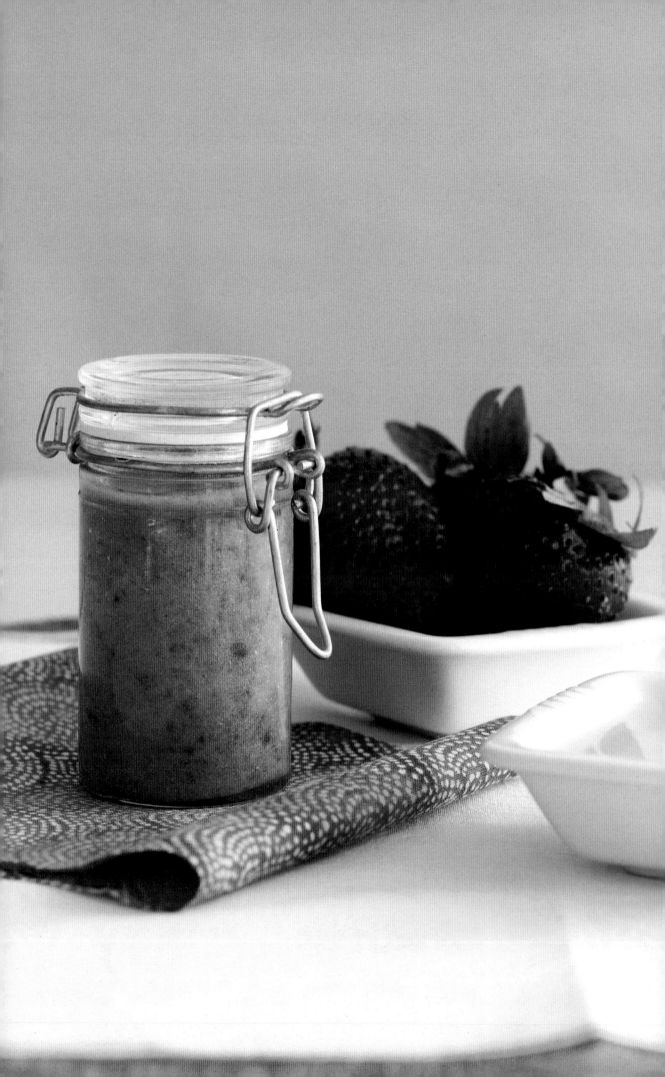

Strawberry Cleanser

I have definitely struggled with my fair share of breakouts and oily teenage skin. This cleanser is my favorite to use during those times. Strawberries contain alpha hydroxy acids, which help exfoliate your skin by removing surface impurities and dead skin cells, leaving you with clearer, smoother skin.

6 whole strawberries

3 tablespoons witch hazel

2 tablespoons almond oil

Put all of the ingredients in a blender and blend until smooth. Pour the cleanser into a clean jar with a tight-fitting lid and store it in the refrigerator, where it will keep for about 2 to 3 weeks.

To use, place a small amount in the palm of your hand, then gently massage it into your skin. Rinse well with warm water, then pat your skin dry.

Yield: 3 ounces

ECO TIP: Use local ingredients and produce when you can. This will support local farms and reduce the amount of fuel needed to transport your ingredients.

Milk Maid Cleanser

This very mild cleanser is great for those with sensitive skin. The baking soda clears away any dead skin buildup, while the milk and egg white nourish and firm the skin. It will give your complexion a wholesome, healthy glow! If you like, you can use the leftover egg yolk to whip up a batch of Pre-Shampoo Hair Conditioner (page 115).

1/2 cup water

1/4 cup whole milk (or soy milk, goat's milk, or hemp milk)

2 tablespoons baking soda

1 egg white

Stir all of the ingredients together until well mixed. Pour the cleanser into a clean container with a tight-fitting lid and store it in the refrigerator, where it will keep for 2 to 3 weeks.

To use, pour a small amount onto a clean, wet washcloth and gently massage it into your face and neck. Rinse well with warm water, then pat your skin dry.

Yield: 7 ounces

Cereal Cleansing Grains

We all know that eating whole grains is good for you, but did you know that your morning whole grain cereal can also nourish your skin from the outside? Oatmeal, cornmeal, and wheat germ are all full of healthy vitamins and minerals, and with their gritty texture they clean and refresh your skin, leaving it smoother and brighter, which is a great way to start your day! Exfoliation is one of the most important parts of skin care, and this simple scrub is one of my favorites for doing the job. I always keep a small jar of this rustic cleanser on hand and use it whenever my complexion looks a bit dull.

2 tablespoons rolled oats
2 tablespoons cornmeal
2 teaspoons wheat germ

Stir all of the ingredients together until well mixed, then store it in an airtight container.

To use, combine 1 or 2 teaspoons of the mixture with an equal amount of water to create a paste. Mix in the palm of your hand and massage this paste gently into damp skin. Rinse well with warm water, then pat your skin dry.

Yield: 3 ounces

$HOPPING TIP: Always buy the cheaper rolled oats, rather than quick-cooking oats. You'll save money, and they're just as effective when it come to skin cleaning. Basically, quick-cooking oats are just chopped-up rolled oats, anyway.

Bye-Bye Blackheads Scrub

Blackheads are pesky blemishes that seem to appear out of nowhere. Technically, they are pores blocked by a mix of sebum and dead skin that turns dark due to oxidation. The good news is that baking soda is here to the rescue! It will get rid of the bacteria and dead skin, leaving you glowing and fresh faced. Adding honey, which has cleansing and antibacterial properties, would be a nice variation on this recipe.

1 tablespoon granulated sugar
1 tablespoon baking soda
2 tablespoons water

Stir all of the ingredients together until well mixed.

To use, massage the entire mixture into damp skin and let it sit for a few minutes. Rinse well with warm water, then pat your skin dry.

Yield: 2 ounces

BLEMISHES

Breakouts can happen to anybody in times of excitement and stress. Stress causes the body to create extra adrenal hormones, which increase the skin's production of natural oils—and in turn, the chance of blemishes.

There are two types of blemishes: comedones and papules, or blackheads and whiteheads. When pores become clogged with oil and other debris, such as dead skin cells or dirt, the oil can oxidize, causing a blackhead. If bacteria are introduced, it will become a whitehead. Never pop a pimple, as this may lead to scarring or infection. Instead, gently dissolve the whitehead with a bit of warm salt water, and then dab a bit of honey or tea tree oil on it to kill any germs.

Sweet Sugar Scrub

Whenever I'm traveling and in need of a facial scrub, I always reach for a couple of sugar packets. The only other thing you really need is a little water. Sugar does a great job of exfoliating skin; adding lemon juice, as in this recipe, promotes cell turnover and helps with skin discoloration. Lemon juice is naturally acidic and helps restore your skin's natural level of acidity, which keeps your complexion fresh and clear.

Juice of ½ lemon

1 teaspoon sugar

1 to 2 teaspoons of your favorite cleanser or soap and water

Mix the lemon juice with an equal amount of water. Then, while washing your face with soap, add the sugar to the lather and massage it gently into your skin. Rinse your skin with the diluted lemon juice, then rinse with clean water and pat your skin dry.

Yield: 1 treatment

SUPER SKIN SCRUBBERS

Besides a good cotton washcloth, here is a list of my favorite skin scrubbers. You can use any of them when you wash your face to get it really clean. Simply mix a teaspoon or two of the scrub with water or your favorite cleanser in the palm of your hand. I use an old coffee grinder to grind nuts, grains, and other scrub ingredients.

- ❋ Sugar
- ❋ Ground sunflower seeds
- ❋ Ground rolled oats
- ❋ Blue cornmeal

- ❋ Ground nuts, such as almonds or walnuts
- ❋ Wheat germ
- ❋ Ground dried orange peels

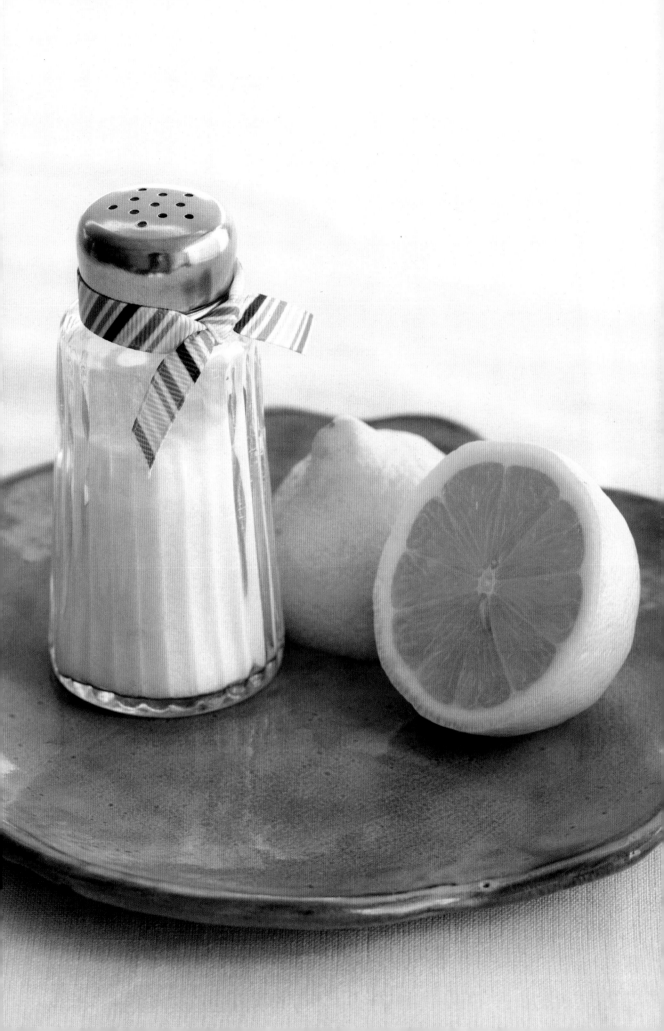

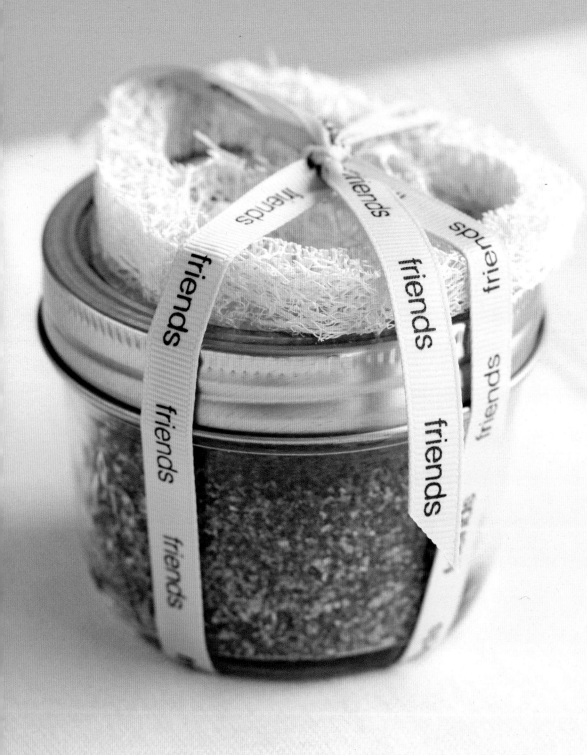

Mermaid Skin Scrub

This scrub is great for ridding your skin of any impurities. You can purchase powdered kelp at any natural food store or Asian food shop, and often it's sold in bulk so you can buy just the amount you need. Seaweed in general is great for the skin. It's full of nutrients and conditioning agents. Plus, it draws toxins away from the skin, explaining why it's become such a popular ingredient for tightening skin or ridding skin of cellulite. It also helps skin retain moisture without adding any oil. I use apple juice in this recipe because it contains pectin, which is soothing to the skin.

¼ **cup powdered kelp**
¼ **cup sugar**
⅓ **cup apple juice**
2 tablespoons honey

Mix the kelp and sugar together, then add the apple juice and honey and stir until well mixed. Spoon the scrub into a clean container with a tight-fitting lid and store it in the refrigerator, where it will keep for 2 to 3 weeks.

To use, massage 1 to 2 teaspoons into your dampened face, then leave it on for 5 minutes. Rinse well with warm water, then pat your skin dry.

Yield: 8 ounces

$HOPPING TIP: ASIAN *SUPER* MARKETS Check out your local Asian market or the Asian food aisle at your grocery store. You can find great deals on dark sesame oil, dried seaweed, adzuki beans (ground up, they make a great skin scrub), wasabi powder, and green tea.

Bunny Love Mask

Carrots are full of carotenes, most importantly beta-carotene, as well as vitamins A and C. Not only are they a nutritional powerhouse, but they can also do great things for your skin. Because beta-carotene is an antioxidant, it can help reduce the effects of too much sun. In addition, the clay in this mask will help strip away impurities and really clean out your pores, leaving you with glowing skin.

¹/₄ cup fresh carrot juice
¹/₄ cup natural clay powder
  (preferably white clay)

Stir the carrot juice and clay together until smooth. For a thicker mask, add a bit more clay. Spoon the mixture into a clean container with a tight-fitting lid and store it in the refrigerator, where it will keep for up to 1 week.

To use, after cleansing, spread about half of the mixture over your face and neck, avoiding the delicate areas around your eyes and mouth. Leave it on for 20 minutes, then rinse well with warm followed by cool water, and pat your skin dry.

Yield: 2 ounces

Fresh Strawberry Mask

This is a great mask for combating acne. Fresh strawberries contain salicylic acid, which is a key ingredient in many over-the-counter acne medications. The strawberries will gently exfoliate your skin and the honey will kill any bad bacteria. Definitely go for this easy mask whenever your skin is troubled and needs some help; you'll also enjoy its fresh berry scent. Use the egg yolk that's left over for a batch of Pre-Shampoo Hair Conditioner (page 115).

¹/₂ cup fresh strawberries
1 egg white
2 teaspoons honey

Put all of the ingredients in a blender and blend on high speed until smooth. Spoon the mixture into a clean container with a tight-fitting lid and store it in the refrigerator, where it will keep for up to 1 week.

To use, after cleansing, spread 1 to 2 tablespoons of the mixture over your face and neck, avoiding the delicate areas around your eyes and mouth. Leave it on for 20 minutes, then rinse well with cool water and pat your skin dry.

Yield: 4 ounces

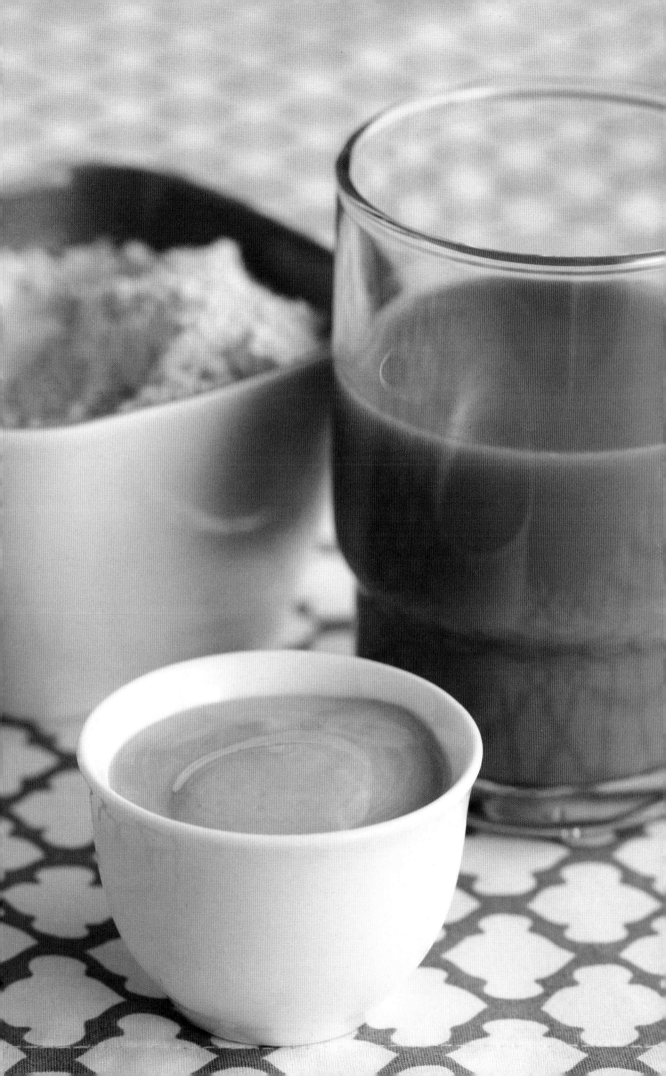

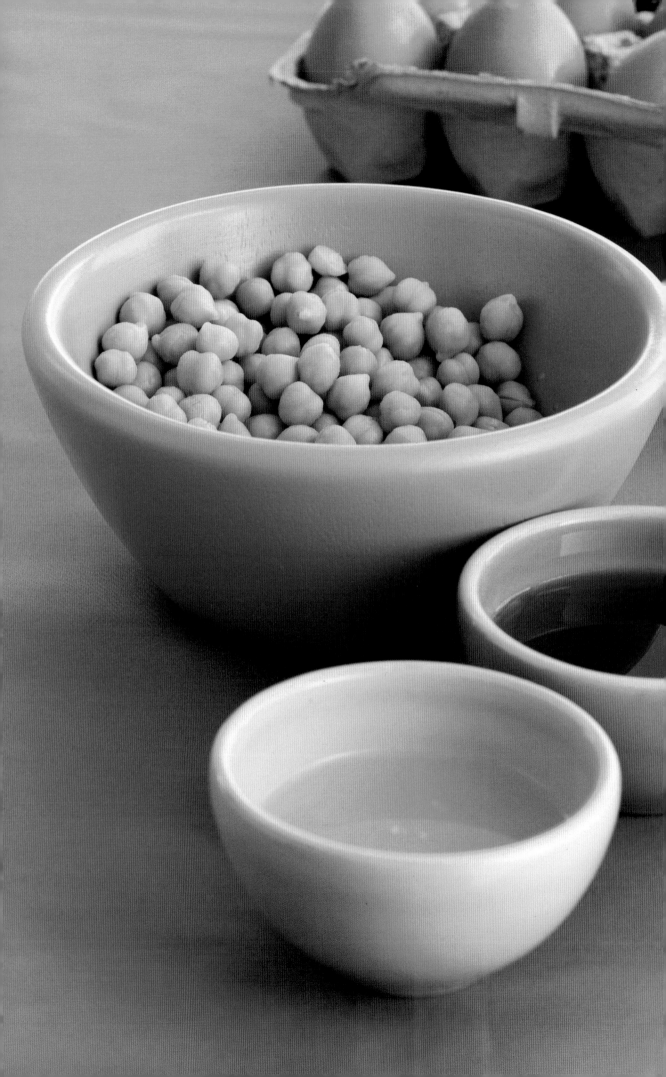

Middle Eastern Hummus Mask

You might want to dip a pita chip into this mask, but don't! It's intended for your skin, not your tummy. This is a great mask for people with dry skin. Both the olive oil and the chickpeas (also known as garbanzo beans) are great for moisturizing the skin and helping it retain moisture. Don't throw the egg white away—draw a Hollywood Bubble Bath (page 66) and relax while the mask works its magic!

¹/₄ cup mashed cooked
  chickpeas
1 teaspoon light olive oil
¹/₄ teaspoon lemon juice
1 egg yolk

Stir all of the ingredients together until you have a smooth paste.

To use, after cleansing, spread the entire mixture over your face and neck, avoiding the delicate areas around your eyes and mouth. Leave it on for 20 minutes, then rinse well with warm water followed by cool water, and pat your skin dry.

Yield: 3 ounces

QUICK TIP: Beaten eggs are a simple and effective facial mask. The part of the egg you use depends on your skin type. For oily skin, use the white; for dry skin, use the yolk, and for normal skin, use the whole egg.

Get-the-Red-Out Facial Mask

Sometimes the skin, especially if it's sensitive, can become irritated and turn an embarrassing shade of red. This soothing mask is great for combating any redness. Its main ingredient is yogurt, which is full of natural fats and proteins that can cool and calm irritated skin.

¹/₄ cup plain whole yogurt
  or sour cream
2 tablespoons honey

Stir the yogurt and honey together until smooth.

To use, after cleansing, spread the entire mixture on your face and neck, avoiding the delicate areas around your eyes and mouth. Leave it on for 15 minutes, then rinse well with warm water and pat your skin dry.

Yield: 3 ounces

Espresso Yourself Facial Mask

I personally like this mask because it contains two of my favorite ingredients: coffee and chocolate. I used to work as a barista at a local coffee stand and one of the most popular drinks was an iced mocha, which provided the inspiration for this cleansing facial mask. The milk and coffee contain naturally occurring acids that help rid your skin of surface debris and dead skin cells, and the cocoa powder helps condition and sooth your complexion. This is a fun mask to give as a gift: Simply package the dry ingredients in a small cellophane bag and place it inside a cute espresso cup or coffee mug. Include directions for mixing the dry ingredients with milk and using the mask. It will definitely perk up your friend's day!

¼ **cup finely ground coffee, preferably espresso roast**
¼ **cup cocoa powder**
½ **cup whole milk**

Stir all of the ingredients together until you have a smooth paste.

To use, after cleansing, spread the entire mixture over your face and neck, avoiding the delicate areas around your eyes and mouth. Leave it on for 15 minutes, then rinse well with warm water and pat your skin dry.

Yield: 4 ounces

GOOD STUFF: COFFEE These days, coffee and caffeine are popular ingredients in skin lotions, creams, masks, and body scrubs. When applied to the skin, coffee is useful as a cleanser and an antioxidant and diuretic. Major cosmetic firms such as Avon, Neutrogena, and L'Oreal have all added caffeine to some of their products. A popular use of ground coffee beans is as a body scrub to reduce cellulite. The caffeine in the coffee dehydrates fat cells by energizing them, which in turn affects the sodium-potassium balance in the cells in a way that allows the cells to eliminate a buildup of excess wastes. The bottom line? Your morning Americano could also slim your thighs!

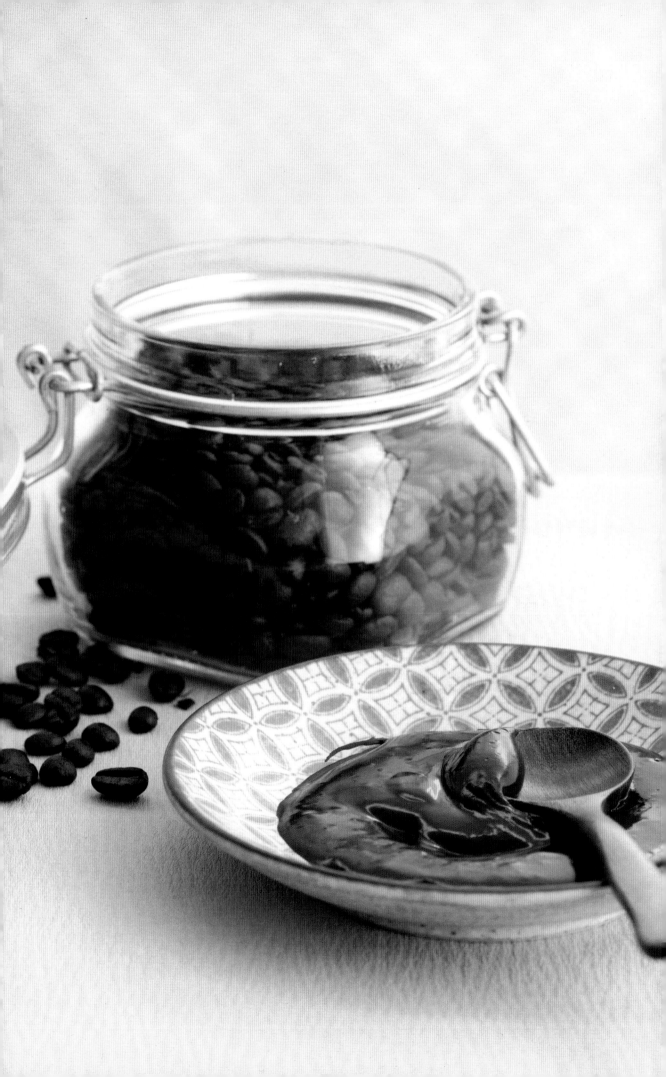

Natural Clay Masks

Clay masks are one of the greatest beauty secrets. Many of the expensive masks you see in department stores are simply variations on a basic clay mask. Because clay extracts impurities from your pores, it will help you maintain clean and clear skin. My personal favorite is French green clay, but I encourage you to experiment with other clays to find your own personal favorite.

2 tablespoons natural clay powder
1 to 2 tablespoons distilled water

Stir the clay and water together until you have a smooth paste.

To use, after cleansing, spread the entire mixture on your face and neck, avoiding the delicate areas around your eyes and mouth. Leave it on for 15 to 20 minutes, until dry. Rinse well with warm water followed by cool water, then pat your skin dry.

Yield: 1 ounce

$HOPPING TIP: CLAY There are many natural clays on the market today. Some are sold in bulk, and others come in bags or jars. They all work basically the same way, providing deep cleansing by drawing out impurities from your pores. Here are a few of the more common clays you'll find. You may have to shop at a natural food store for some of these.

❋ **Fuller's earth:** A fine gray clay that comes from algae in seabeds and river bottoms

❋ **Kaolin or white China clay:** A fine white powder that's abundant across the globe but was named for Kaolin (or Gaoling, meaning "high hill"), in China

❋ **French green clay:** A fine, pale green clay from southern France

❋ **Bentonite:** A white volcanic clay that's especially abundant in the western United States

❋ **Rhassoul mud:** A red clay from the Atlas Mountains in northwest Africa

Blueberry Antioxidant Face Mask

Blueberries are packed with powerful antioxidants. These antioxidants target free radicals, which can wreak havoc on skin cells. By using this mask now, you'll be preventing signs of aging later in life. Trust me; you'll thank yourself down the road! If you can't find fresh blueberries, you can use frozen blueberries in this recipe.

8 to 10 blueberries
1 tablespoon plain yogurt
1 tablespoon lemon juice

Mash or blend the blueberries together with the yogurt and lemon juice.

To use, after cleansing, spread the entire mixture over your face and neck, avoiding the delicate areas around your eyes and mouth. Leave it on for 15 minutes, then rinse well with warm water and pat your skin dry.

Yield: 2 ounces

Smoothing and Softening Face Mask

This face mask is a natural choice when your skin needs an energizing pick-me-up. Goat's milk is great for rejuvenating and moisturizing skin, which is why it's so widely used in skin care products. And the rice flour in this recipe is great for combating skin problems and smoothing your complexion. Look for both ingredients in natural food stores or well-stocked grocery stores.

¼ cup rice flour
2 tablespoons honey
2 tablespoons goat's milk

Stir all of the ingredients together until well mixed. Spoon the mixture into a clean container with a tight-fitting lid and store it in the refrigerator, where it will keep for about 2 weeks.

To use, after cleansing, spread about 1 tablespoon of the mask over your face and neck, avoiding the delicate areas around your eyes and mouth. Leave it on for 15 minutes, then rinse well with warm water and pat your skin dry.

Yield: 3 ounces

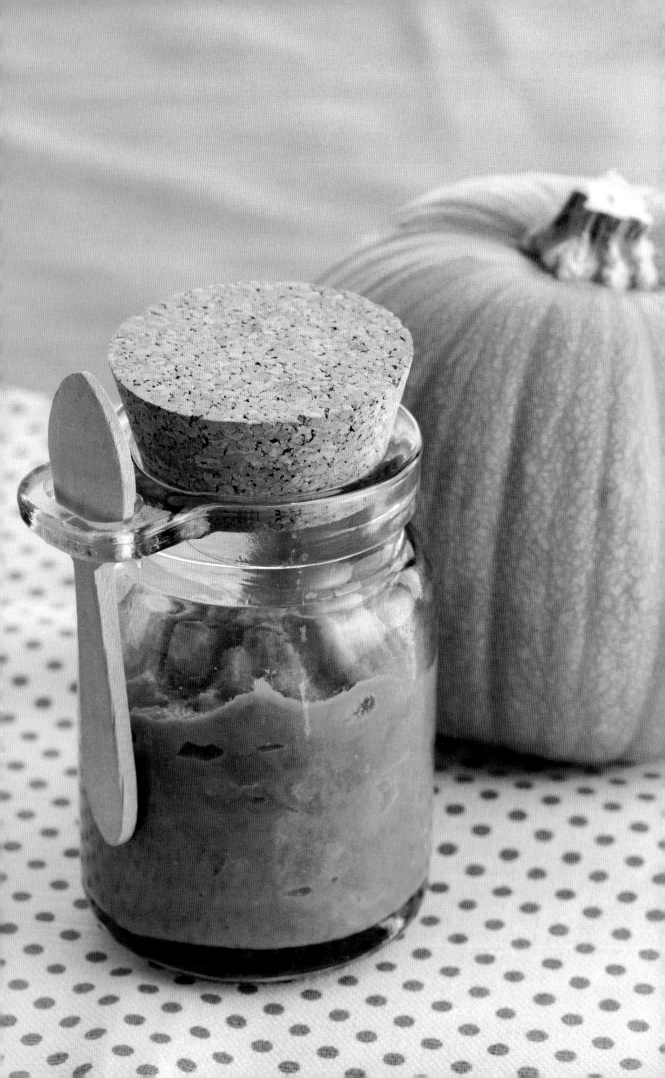

Pumpkin Pie Mask

My favorite holiday dessert is pumpkin pie. Pumpkin is very nourishing to the skin. It contains powerful antioxidants as well as alpha hydroxy acids, so it sloughs off dead skin while protecting the underlying layer and helping it retain moisture. This is a great mask for the fall and winter months, when your skin may need some good exfoliation and protection from the cold weather. Plus, it makes a fun Halloween or Thanksgiving gift. Package it in a small jar with a simple bow and a small note of thanks. It's perishable, so store it in the refrigerator and tell the person who receives it to do the same.

¼ cup canned pumpkin puree
2 tablespoons vanilla yogurt
   or sour cream
1 tablespoon honey

Stir all of the ingredients together until you have a smooth paste. Spoon the mask into a clean container with a tight-fitting lid and store it in the refrigerator, where it will keep for about 2 weeks.

To use, after cleansing, spread 1 tablespoon of the mask over your face and neck, avoiding the delicate areas around your eyes and mouth. Leave it on for 15 minutes, then rinse well with warm water and pat your skin dry.

Yield: 3½ ounces

Charcoal Face Mask

Charcoal is definitely an unexpected beauty ingredient. However, activated charcoal works wonders to deeply cleanse pores. The tea tree oil makes this mask clarifying, but it's definitely strong and shouldn't be used on sensitive skin. That said, if you suffer with blackheads, you should definitely give this mask a try. Don't be alarmed that this mask is so black in color; the results are worth it. Just make sure you rinse well after using this mask so that you remove all traces of the black charcoal from your pores and skin.

2 teaspoons distilled water
2 teaspoons powdered activated charcoal (5 to 6 capsules)
2 to 3 drops tea tree oil

Stir the water into the charcoal until it forms a paste, then stir in the tea tree oil.

To use, after cleansing, spread the entire mixture over your face and neck, avoiding the delicate areas around your eyes and mouth. Leave it on for 10 minutes, then thoroughly wash it off with warm water and pat your skin dry.

Yield: ³/₄ ounce

$HOPPING TIP: CHARCOAL Activated charcoal is simply burnt wood that has been processed to increase its surface area and make it more porous. This is usually done by the addition of gases such as oxygen, carbon dioxide, or steam. This activation process creates a very absorbent material that's used for a variety of purposes, including removing toxins from the body, and especially from the digestive system. You can find activated charcoal at the drugstore or in the health care section of the grocery store. It's sold in powdered and capsule form. If you can only find the capsules, that's fine—just break them open! Many cosmetics firms are now adding charcoal to their facial masks to help remove toxins and calm irritated skin.

Old-Fashioned Astringent

Pure witch hazel is a classic astringent that has been used for generations. I remember my own great-grandmother using it daily, along with sweet-smelling rose water, to keep her skin soft and clean. Used straight, witch hazel can be harsh and drying, so it's a good idea to dilute it with water, as in this recipe. Not all skin types require an astringent; however, if you suffer from oily or acne-prone skin, daily use of this astringent is a good idea. Use it after cleansing your skin and before moisturizing.

3 tablespoons distilled water
3 tablespoons rose water
1 tablespoon witch hazel

Pour all of the ingredients into a clean bottle with a tight-fitting lid and shake to combine.

To use, apply the astringent to your skin using a clean cotton ball.

Yield: 3¹/₂ ounces

BEAUTY SMARTS: WHAT DID WOMEN USE BEFORE THERE WAS A COSMETICS INDUSTRY? Homemade body care products date back to ancient times. Women have always been very resourceful in treating their skin and hair and finding ways to look their best, and many of the treatments we use today have withstood the test of time. Cleopatra bathed in milk to soothe and soften her skin, pioneer women used sugar to kill bacteria and cleanse their skin, the early Pilgrims stained their lips with berries, and the Mayans used cocoa butter as a skin moisturizer. I guess it shows that there's no such thing as a new idea; just improved-upon ideas. If you take a good look at the body care products available today, you can see for yourself that they're stocked with milk baths, sugar scrubs, lipsticks, and body butters.

Powerful Pomegranate Toner

Pomegranates have been a symbol of beauty and goodness since ancient times. The juice is a powerful antioxidant that does great things for skin. It's especially useful for those with combination skin, as it isn't too drying and also promotes the regeneration of skin cells. I often use bottled pomegranate juice because it is available year-round, but you can also make your own fresh juice. An easy way to extract the seeds from a pomegranate is to submerge the whole fruit in a bowl of cold water as you peel it. The seeds will float to the top. Place a cup of seeds into a strainer over a bowl and gently press on them with a large spoon to release the juice.

¼ cup pomegranate juice
3 tablespoons witch hazel
2 tablespoons distilled water

Pour all of the ingredients into a clean bottle with a tight-fitting lid and shake to combine. To extend the shelf life, you may store this toner in the refrigerator, where it will keep for 2 to 3 weeks.

To use, apply the toner to your face using a clean cotton ball.

Yield: 4½ ounces

Bee Happy Toner

Toners are less harsh on the skin than astringents because they typically contain less alcohol. This is a great toner for anyone with normal to oily skin. The honey adds an antibacterial property, and the lemon juice helps even out skin tone. Because of the honey, this toner may feel slightly sticky at first, but the stickiness tends to disappear after the solution sits.

1 tablespoon honey
2 tablespoons witch hazel
1 tablespoon rose water or
   distilled water
1 teaspoon lemon juice

Pour all of the ingredients into a clean bottle with a tight-fitting lid and shake to combine.

To use, apply the toner to your face using a clean cotton ball.

Yield: 2 ounces

ECO TIP: When applying astringents and toners, use organic cotton pads and balls. Commercial cotton is heavily sprayed with pesticides and other chemicals. Choose organic cotton to cut down on the use of harmful chemicals and help the environment.

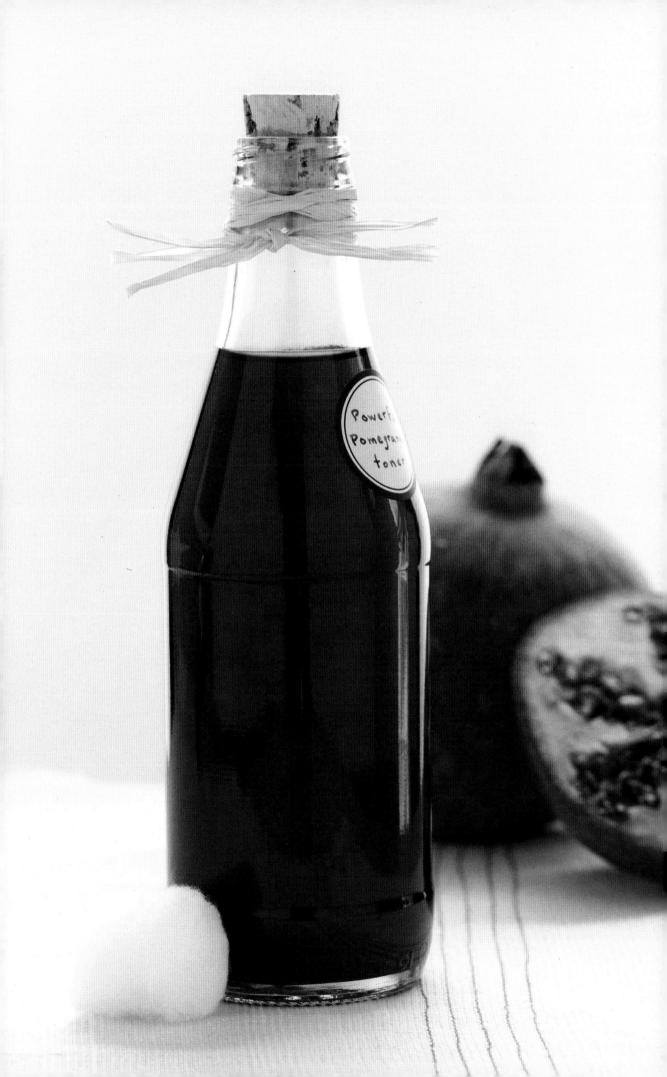

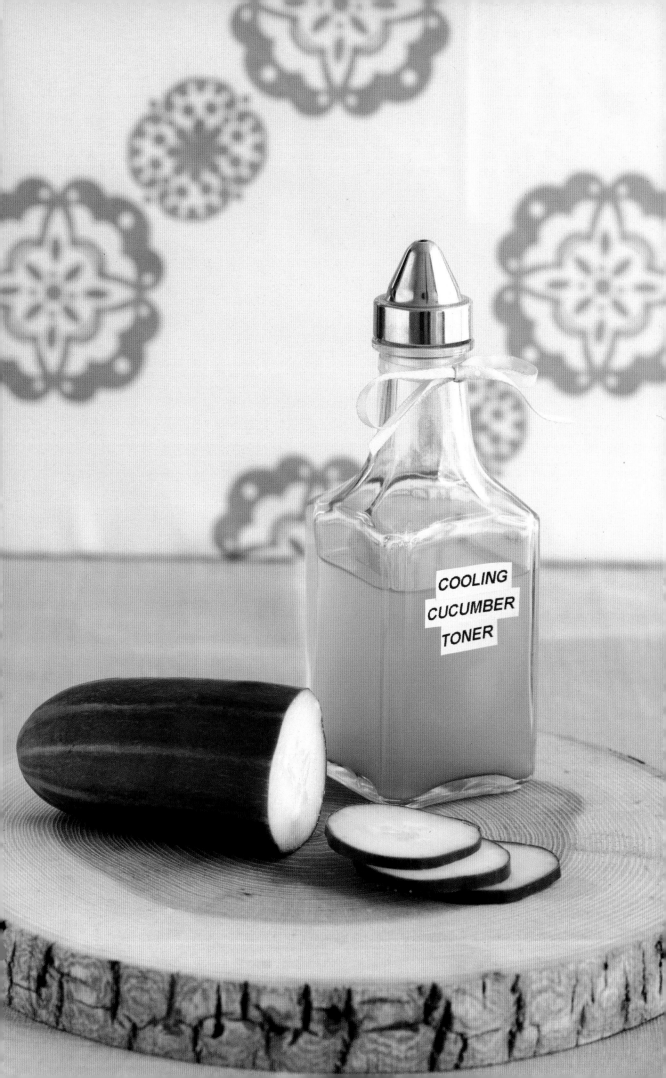

COOLING
CUCUMBER
TONER

Cooling Cucumber Toner

This toner is very mild and works well for all skin types. Cucumber is great for soothing and softening skin because it has the same pH as healthy skin. If you ever wake up feeling like your face is a little puffy, this toner is your best bet for calming and tightening your skin.

½ cucumber with peel, chopped
3 tablespoons witch hazel
2 tablespoons distilled water

Put all of the ingredients in a blender or food processor and blend until smooth. Pour the mixture through a fine-mesh sieve to remove all of the solids, then pour the toner into a clean bottle with a tight-fitting lid. Store this toner in the refrigerator for a longer shelf life—it should last for several weeks.

To use, apply the toner to your face using a clean cotton ball.

Yield: 4½ ounces

QUICK TIP: A classic home beauty trick is to use fresh cucumber slices to soothe puffy eyes. Simply lie down, close your eyes, put a cucumber slice on each, and let this naturally astringent and cooling vegetable work its magic.

Lemonade Toner

Fresh lemon juice makes a great toner for the skin, but it should always be diluted since it's too acidic to use straight on most skin types. It can even out skin tone and help fade any discoloration. It will also clean out your pores and get your skin really clean. After using this toner, follow up with a light natural oil, such as light sesame oil or almond oil, since lemon juice can be drying.

¼ cup lemon juice
3 tablespoons witch hazel
2 tablespoons distilled water

Pour all of the ingredients into a clean bottle with a tight-fitting lid and shake to combine.

To use, apply the toner to your face using a clean cotton ball.

Yield: 4½ ounces

Not Your Grandmother's Toner

My grandmother loves the scent of lavender, but this gentle toner isn't just for her generation; it's something girls of all ages can enjoy. I love to use floral waters on my face after cleansing because they're so mild and refreshing. Put this toner in a clean spray bottle and spray it on your face (eyes closed!).

¼ cup rose water
¼ cup lavender water
3 tablespoons witch hazel

Pour all of the ingredients into a clean bottle with a tight-fitting lid and shake to combine.

To use, apply the toner to your face using a clean cotton ball.

Yield: 5½ ounces

$HOPPING TIP: FLORAL WATERS You may have to search a bit for scented floral waters. I've found them at the grocery store in the skin care aisle, and also in the mixers aisle, since they're sometimes used for creating scented drinks. You may also be able to find them at specialty import stores and ethnic markets. Greek and Persian markets often have several types of rose water, orange flower water, chamomile water, and borage flower water at resonable prices. If you want to make your own scented waters, add a few drops of your favorite floral essential oil to a cup of distilled water. Some of my favorite floral scents are frangipani (plumeria), ylang-ylang, lavender, and jasmine. You can find essential oils at many natural food stores in the body care section.

Fresh Parsley Skin Toner

This skin pick-me-up will leave you feeling very refreshed. Parsley promotes circulation, and it also has antiseptic qualities that make it purifying and cleansing. This toner is ideal for anyone who suffers from acne and also has sensitive skin.

1 cup water
½ cup chopped parsley

Bring the water to a boil. Place the parsley in a clean, heatproof bowl and pour in the boiling water. Allow the mixture to cool completely, then strain through a fine-mesh sieve and pour into a clean bottle with a tight-fitting lid. Store any leftover toner in the refrigerator; it should keep for a few weeks.

To use, apply the toner to your face using a clean cotton ball.

Yield: 8 ounces

Australian Tea Tree Toner

When I was two, my family lived in Australia. Of course I wasn't into making my own cosmetics at that time, but my mom tells me that she used a variety of Aussie concoctions on me. One of the skin secrets you quickly pick up there is the magic of tea tree oil. On a recent trip to Australia I brought home several bottles of the clean, strongly scented oil. Fortunately, you don't have to travel Down Under to take advantage of this wonder oil; it's readily available in the skin care section of many natural food stores and drugstores. You can use this toner no matter what your skin type, but it's especially effective for problematic or acne-prone skin.

¼ **cup distilled water**
¼ **cup witch hazel**
1 **teaspoon tea tree oil**

Pour all of the ingredients into a clean bottle with a tight-fitting lid and shake to combine.

To use, apply the toner to your face using a clean cotton ball.

Yield: 4 ounces

GOOD STUFF: ESSENTIAL OILS Have you ever noticed that when you peel an orange, it often releases a fine mist of pure citrus scent and natural oils? That oil is what is known as an essential oil. Essential oils are highly concentrated aromatic extracts of different plants. They come in a wide variety of scents, ranging from the common, such as lemon, orange, and peppermint, to the more exotic, such as ylang-ylang, patchouli, and sandalwood. They also vary in cost based on how difficult they are to produce. You'll find bottles of various essential oils at many bath and body boutiques, natural food stores, and some grocery stores. They come in small bottles and may seem expensive, but the scents are so highly concentrated that you usually use only a drop or two, so they last a long time.

Aromatherapy is the practice of using scents to alter your mood or even your health, and essential oils are an important part of this practice. Knowingly or not, you may already have experienced this ancient practice by using lavender-scented bath salts to relax or by using a peppermint massage oil to energize your body and mind. **Because essential oils are so concentrated, you should always dilute them and never apply them directly to the skin.** Some may cause a rash or reaction, even if they're diluted. If you're using an essential oil for the first time and aren't sure how you'll react, mix a few drops in some natural oil and apply it to a spot on your body that won't show, such as the back of your leg or arm. If you don't have a reaction within a few hours, it's probably safe for you to use. If you do experience a reaction, it's always best to consult you doctor and to avoid using that particular oil in the future. Also, because essential oils are so highly concentrated, it's never a good idea to ingest them. If you use them in a treatment on your face, avoid your eye and mouth area to be safe.

Green Tea Toner

For me, green tea is more than the perfect drink; it's also great for my skin. I've made this simple, inexpensive toner for several years now, and it's a key part of my everyday skin care routine. In fact, during the summer, I keep a small spray bottle full of this toner in my bag to refresh my complexion throughout the day. Green tea is a powerful antioxidant because it's rich in polyphenols, chemicals that help slow down damage to your skin from the environment. There are plenty of different brands of green tea to choose from, and they all work equally well. To save money, you can use loose tea leaves when brewing up this toner.

½ cup distilled water

1 to 2 green tea bags, or 2 teaspoons green tea leaves

Bring the water to a boil. Place the tea in a clean, heatproof bowl and pour in the boiling water. Steep for 2 to 3 minutes, then remove the tea bags or strain out the tea leaves and allow the liquid to cool before pouring it into a clean bottle with a tight-fitting lid.

To use, apply the toner to your face using a clean cotton ball.

Yield: 4 ounces

QUICK TIPS: Besides being a skin toner, green tea can also be used as a refreshing facial treatment at the end of a long day. Simply soak a cotton washcloth in cool green tea, then place it over your face for ten minutes. Additionally, you can reduce under-eye puffiness and soothe tired eyes by placing two cold, used caffeinated tea bags (such as orange pekoe or black) over your eyes for ten to fifteen minutes.

GOOD STUFF: TEA If you walk down the tea aisle at your grocery store, you'll be amazed at how many choices you have. More than just a beverage, tea has become a "hot" ingredient in natural cosmetics these days, and many major cosmetics companies have entire product lines featuring tea. Tea is a strong antioxidant rich in vitamins C and E, and research shows it to be a powerful enemy of damaging free radicals, which cause our bodies to age. It has a variety of benefits and can be used all over your body to cleanse your skin, soothe sunburn, highlight your hair, relax your muscles, and soothe puffy eyes. All true teas come from the same plant (*Camellia sinensis*); the difference between different types, such as green, oolong, white, and black, has to do with the way the leaves are dried and treated. Herbal teas aren't true teas; they're made from the dried leaves and flowers of other plants. Don't think of herbal teas as the same as regular tea. They have their own unique properties. For example, chamomile tea is very relaxing, whereas peppermint tea will calm an upset stomach and energize your body.

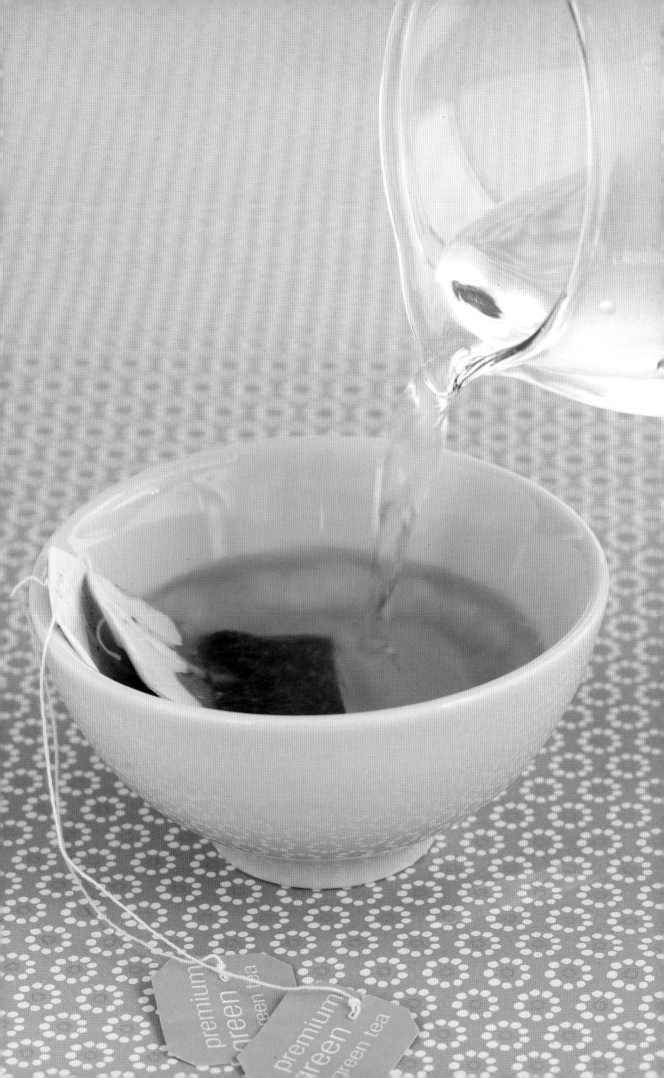

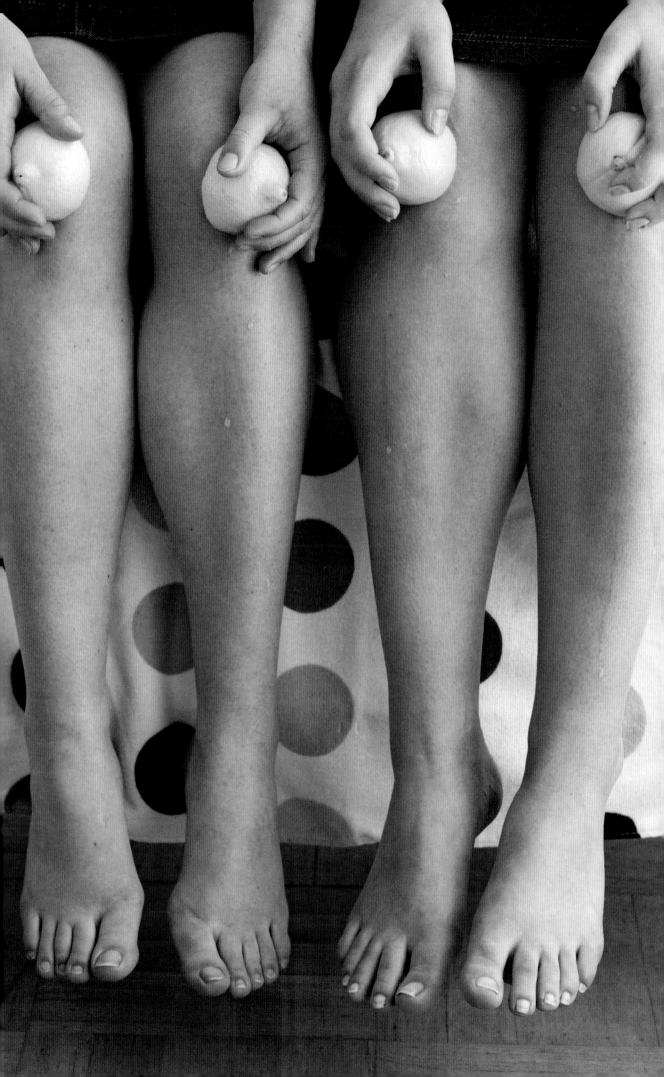

FOR THE BODY

The skin is the largest organ of the body. It protects us, enhances our sense of touch, and helps control our body temperature. Keeping the body full of water is another important function of the skin. In fact, dry skin isn't necessarily a sign of loss of skin oils, as is commonly thought—it can simply be a sign of loss of water from the body. Skin needs water to stay looking healthy and be flexible, and loss of water from our skin makes it look dry and older than it should. That's why it's important to use a good natural oil, body cream, or lotion to form a protective layer, which will prevent water from evaporating from the skin.

Moisturizing after bathing or showering and while your body is still a little damp is a great way to lock in moisture and help prevent dry skin.

I like to think of skin as being its own ecosystem or environment. To be healthy, skin must maintain a delicate balance between good bacteria, microorganisms, and yeast, as well as the right level of acidity, which is why you'll see some skin products claiming to restore pH levels. The skin is naturally acidic, which keeps it healthy and helps it combat surface pollutants, which are primarily alkaline, and therefore are neutralized by the acidity of skin. Washing your skin with strong soap can interfere with its pH bacteria balance, which then needs to be restored. A simple after-bath spray of diluted apple cider vinegar or green tea will easily do the trick.

There are several ways to take good care of your skin. Of course, the beauty basics that apply to your face are also appropriate for your whole body: keep your skin clean, full of moisture, and protected from the sun. I cannot overstress how important sun protection is for your skin—and please stay out of those tanning machines. The FDA regularly issues warnings about this, going so far as to say "There is no such thing as a safe tan." Plus, skin that looks like a leather handbag is just not cool.

The skin on the body is generally thicker than that on the face, so it can handle stronger products and ingredients. In most cases, tropical fruit acids, salt scrubs, and heavier oils that are too much for your face can be applied to your body.

Massage oils, bath products, and shower gels are all easy to make and fun to use. They also help cleanse, tone, and moisturize your skin. I sometimes shower twice a day, especially if I've had a good workout at the gym, so dry skin can be a problem. I like to use vegetable-based soaps or soaps made with natural oils, since they help keep my skin hydrated and smooth. Additionally, it is always a good idea to follow up after any skin care treatment with a light moisturizer or natural oil.

Exfoliating is important for healthy skin all over your body, not just on your face. It's a good idea to use a natural loofah sponge, body brush, scrub, or other exfoliant weekly to help remove dead skin cells, boost circulation, and aid your lymphatic system in ridding your body of waste. Plus, exfoliation will soften and smooth your

SLIP, SLOP, SLAP

In Australia, the government has a public service campaign about sun safety with a goofy but completely catchy slogan: "Slip, Slop, Slap." This is short for slip on a T-shirt, slop on some sunscreen, and slap on a hat. Silly? Yes, but it's easy to remember and has been very effective in reducing the number of cases of skin cancer.

skin. You might have noticed that your skin changes when the seasons change; this is another good time for a full body scrub. After a full summer of sun and fun, my body needs a thorough overall exfoliation before I head back to school.

I also like to do home spa treatments on the weekends. I devote an entire afternoon to pampering my body and relaxing.

All you need are some fluffy towels, your favorite tunes, some magazines, and high-quality natural ingredients. I've included some of my favorite spa treatments in this section—your skin will thank you, as will your frame of mind. You only have one body, so take good care of it. I know that when I do, I feel happier and healthier!

TEN TIPS FOR HEALTHY SKIN

Here are ten simple things you can do to keep your body happy and healthy, which will do wonders for keeping your skin healthy:

1. **Move:** Walk, run, dance, or find some other way to exercise every day.

2. **De-stress:** When you're stressed-out, your body produces hormones that can lead to breakouts and, over time, damage your skin cells and your overall health. Plan a quiet time for yourself every day.

3. **Practice safe sun:** Use sunscreen every day and cover up when you're outdoors. And don't forget to bust out that stylish broad-rimmed hat.

4. **Moisturize:** Lock moisture into your skin after bathing or showering.

5. **Eat healthy:** Nosh on a balanced diet full of fresh fruits and vegetables and healthy, high-quality protein.

6. **Exfoliate:** Once a week, buff away dead cells and surface debris that can clog your pores.

7. **Smooth:** Treat those typical rough skin spots, such as knees, elbows, and heels, to some extra pampering.

8. **Scent:** Use fragrance and natural scents to energize, focus, or calm down.

9. **Soothe sore muscles:** Massage your whole body or soak in a relaxing bath.

10. **Celebrate:** Feeling good about your body and life, and loving yourself and your life will show!

Healthy Hemp Massage Oil

Hemp oil is great for overall well-being. It's rich in vitamin E and omega-3s, the good fats we're hearing so much about these days. I like to use it like flax oil, as a light, skin-nourishing oil to help soften dry skin, leaving it smooth and healthy. It's especially nice to use in the winter months, when everyone needs more moisture because of indoor heating systems and colder air outdoors, which both dry out the skin and hair. And because hemp oil has anti-inflammatory properties, it's a perfect base for massage oil for sore muscles. This oil makes a great gift for anyone who's active in sports and could use a bit of pampering. Package it in a cool bottle and label it with a digital photo of your friend in action.

½ cup hemp oil

1 teaspoon vitamin E oil

1 tablespoon fresh herbs, such as basil, lavender, rosemary, or mint, or a combination

Mix all of the ingredients together in a microwave-safe container or in a small saucepan. Gently heat the mixture in the microwave or on the stove, but don't let it come to a boil. Pour the warm oil through a fine-mesh sieve to remove any bits of herbs, then let it cool completely before spooning it into a clean jar.

To use, massage a small amount into your skin.

Yield: 4 ounces

GOOD STUFF: IT'S HIP TO USE HEMP! Hemp oil is getting to be super popular because it's an effective moisturizer even though it has a light feel. It can be used by all skin types, and because it doesn't clog your pores, it's good for acne-prone skin. My only complaint about this wonder oil is its mildly nutty scent. It takes a bit of getting used to when used straight on your skin or hair, but some people actually enjoy the scent.

Hemp is often confused with marijuana, as it comes from the same plant, but don't worry, it's perfectly legal and doesn't contain any THC, the compound that produces psychoactive effects. Many states have passed laws allowing growers to produce and sell hemp products, and many companies are starting to feature hemp products. In fact, the hemp line produced by the Body Shop is one of their best sellers. Hemp oil is found at many natural food stores. Some people even take a teaspoon or two daily to help them get their essential fatty acids.

Ultimate Body Butter

I love moisturizing with a thick lotion or body butter, as it does the best job at keeping skin soft and well moisturized. This recipe is packed with moisturizing oils, so if your skin is looking at all dull or flaky, this is definitely the cure for you.

1/4 cup grated cocoa butter
2 tablespoons light sesame oil
1 tablespoon coconut oil
1 tablespoon avocado oil
1 tablespoon grated beeswax

Combine all of the ingredients in an ovenproof glass container. Place the container into a pan with a 1 to 2 inch water bath. Melt the oils and wax gently. Place all of the ingredients in a microwave-safe container or on the stovetop in a double boiler. Microwave on low heat for short intervals, stirring occasionally, just until the ingredients are melted; if using a double boiler, stir frequently and remove from the heat as soon as the ingredients are melted. Stir until the ingredients are well mixed. Pour the mixture into a clean jar with a tight-fitting lid and stir it again once it's cool. Store it in a cool, dry spot, where it will keep for 4 to 6 weeks.

To use, spread the butter on your body and massage into your skin.

Yield: 4 ounces

Chocolate Massage Butter

I'm a full-fledged chocoholic—in fact, I have emergency chocolate stashes all over my dorm room. This rich body butter has the yummy scent of chocolate without any of the calories. It can be used as a moisturizer as well as a massage oil. Just rub some in your hands to warm it up and you'll have a massage oil and a chocolaty snack for the senses, all in one!

1/4 **cup grated cocoa butter**
1 **tablespoon grated dark chocolate**
2 **tablespoons light sesame oil**
1 **tablespoon light olive oil**
1 **tablespoon grated beeswax**

Place all of the ingredients in a microwave-safe container or on the stovetop in a double boiler. Microwave on low heat for short intervals, stirring occasionally, just until the ingredients are melted; if using a double boiler, stir frequently and remove from the heat as soon as the ingredients are melted. Stir until the ingredients are well mixed, then pour the hot liquid into a clean container, or for small individual bars, pour it into an ice cube tray and let it cool completely.

To use, either rub the entire massage butter bar over your skin, or warm and soften a bit of the massage butter by rubbing it between your hands, then massage it into clean skin.

Yield: 4 ounces

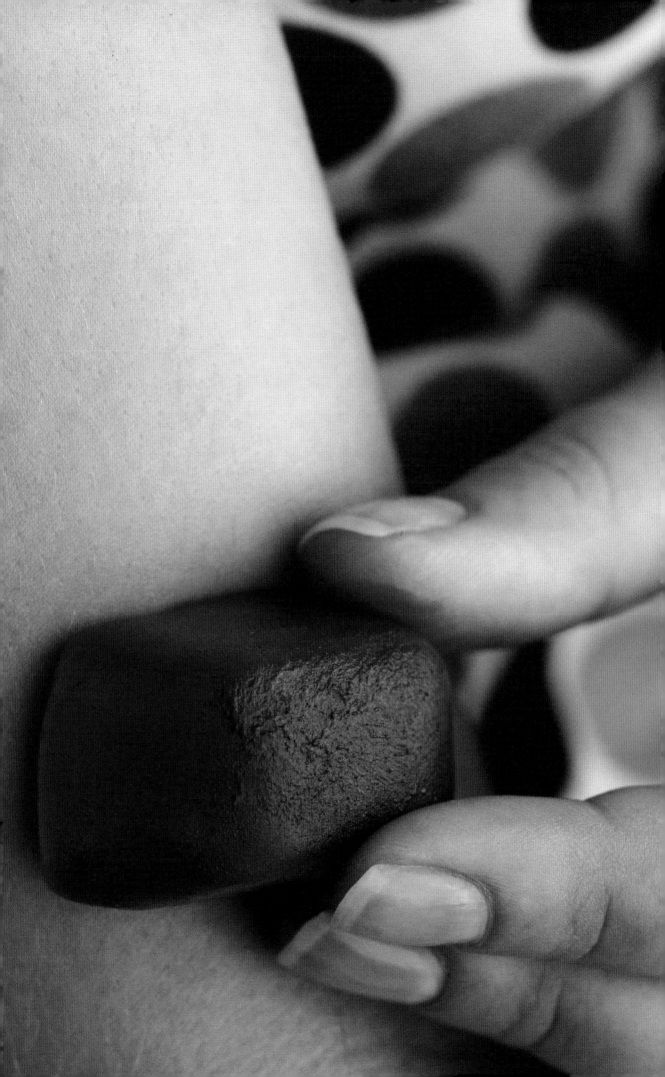

African Shea Butter Lotion

Shea butter is an ivory-colored natural fat that comes from African shea trees and is used much like cocoa butter. In cosmetics, it acts as a moisturizer and emollient and also has anti-inflammatory properties. Shea butter can treat all types of skin conditions, from scars to chapped lips, and is useful in treating acne because it is nongreasy and easily absorbed by the skin. It provides mild UV protection from the sun but it is not a replacement for your sunscreen (its SPF is probably around 6). It can be found in natural food stores in the skin care section.

1/2 cup boiling water
1/8 teaspoon borax powder
1/2 cup almond oil
1 tablespoon grated shea butter

Bring the water to a boil. Place the borax powder in a clean, heatproof bowl, pour in the boiling water, and stir well. Set aside. Place the oil and shea butter in a microwave-safe container, mix together, and microwave on high heat for 1 minute, until the shea butter is melted. If it has not all melted yet, you can stir the oil until it does. Pour the oil mixture into a blender or food processor and blend on low speed, adding the hot water mixture in a slow, steady stream. Blend on high speed until well mixed. You should have a milky white lotion. Pour the mixture into a clean container to cool.

To use, massage into your skin.

Yield: 4 ounces

Energizing Leg Gel

Move, jump, run, and dance . . . after using this energizing leg gel, that is! This recipe is the perfect pick-me-up at the end of a busy day. Peppermint oil is a well-known energizer, and when combined with the aloe and witch hazel, it makes for an elixir that will instantly wake up any slow or tired muscles. This is a light, nongreasy recipe, so you can use it throughout the day whenever your legs need a quick boost. It makes a great gift for an active friend.

1/2 cup aloe vera gel
1 tablespoon witch hazel
1 1/2 teaspoons cornstarch
3 to 4 drops peppermint oil

Combine the aloe vera, witch hazel, and cornstarch in a microwave-safe container or on the stovetop in a double boiler. Microwave on high heat for 1 to 2 minutes, stirring every 30 seconds; if using a double boiler, cook, stirring occasionally, for about 5 minutes. Stir until the ingredients are well mixed, then allow the mixture to cool. Add the peppermint oil and stir thoroughly, then pour into a clean container with a tight-fitting lid. Store it in a cool, dry, dark spot, where it will keep for 3 to 4 weeks.

To use, massage the gel into your legs and feet for an instant cooling sensation.

Yield: 4 1/2 ounces

Maui Pineapple Body Scrub

Whenever I eat a fresh pineapple, I always save the peel to use as body scrubbers—a trick I learned while on vacation in Hawaii. Use the inner part of the peel, not the outside, which would be very ouchy. Fresh pineapple contains an active enzyme called bromelain, which acts as an effective natural exfoliator and will leave your skin super smooth and clean. Your body will say *mahalo* (thank you)! The peel from $1/4$ pineapple is about the right amount for a whole body treatment; wrap up the rest of the peel and store it in the refrigerator or freezer to use another time.

The peel of $1/4$ of a fresh pineapple, cut into 3- to 4-inch-wide strips
Coarse salt or sugar (optional)

Sprinkle the inside of the pineapple peels with salt or sugar for extra exfoliating power, if you like.

To use, stand in the shower or tub and scrub your skin with the inside of the pineapple peels just like you'd use a sponge or loofah to scrub your body and exfoliate dead skin cells. Rinse well afterward.

Yield: 1 whole body treatment

GOOD STUFF: NATURAL FRUIT ENZYMES Fruit enzymes are a popular beauty ingredient because they quickly cleanse and soften the skin. Papaya contains papain, pineapple contains bromelain, kiwifruit has actinidin, and figs are rich in ficin. These enzymes are well suited for smoothing out typical rough skin spots, such as the elbows, knees, and feet, but I don't recommend using them on your face, as they may be too harsh. You'll see many commercial body scrubs and treatments containing these superfoods because they are so effective.

Chocolate Walnut Body Polish

This body scrub sounds good enough to eat, but it's actually a dessert for your skin. Weekly exfoliation is important for healthy skin, and this particular recipe is perfect for dry skin that could use a bit more oil or moisturizing. Be forewarned: It's always a good idea to eat dessert before you use body care products that smell good enough to eat!

½ cup raw sugar

¼ cup walnut oil

1 tablespoon finely chopped walnuts

1 tablespoon cocoa powder

Stir all of the ingredients together until well mixed. Spoon the scrub into a clean jar with a tight-fitting lid and store it in a cool, dry location, where it will keep for about 4 weeks.

To use, stand in the shower or tub and massage the body polish into damp skin. Rinse well afterward.

Yield: 7 ounces

Soy Body Scrub

Soy is great for the skin. It increases collagen production and helps keep skin tone even. This scrub provides those benefits while also including sugar for exfoliation and vegetable oil for moisturizing to produce healthy, fresh skin. Soy milk is easy to find at most any grocery store and comes in various flavors, which are fun to experiment with in this recipe.

¼ cup sugar

2 tablespoons vegetable oil

2 tablespoons soy milk

Stir all of the ingredients together until you have a smooth cream. Spoon the scrub into a clean jar with a tight-fitting lid and store it in the refrigerator, where it will keep for about 2 weeks.

To use, stand in the shower or tub before bathing and gently massage the mixture all over your body to increase circulation and remove any dry or flaky skin. Rinse well, then be sure to use a good moisturizer or light natural oil afterward.

Yield: 4 ounces

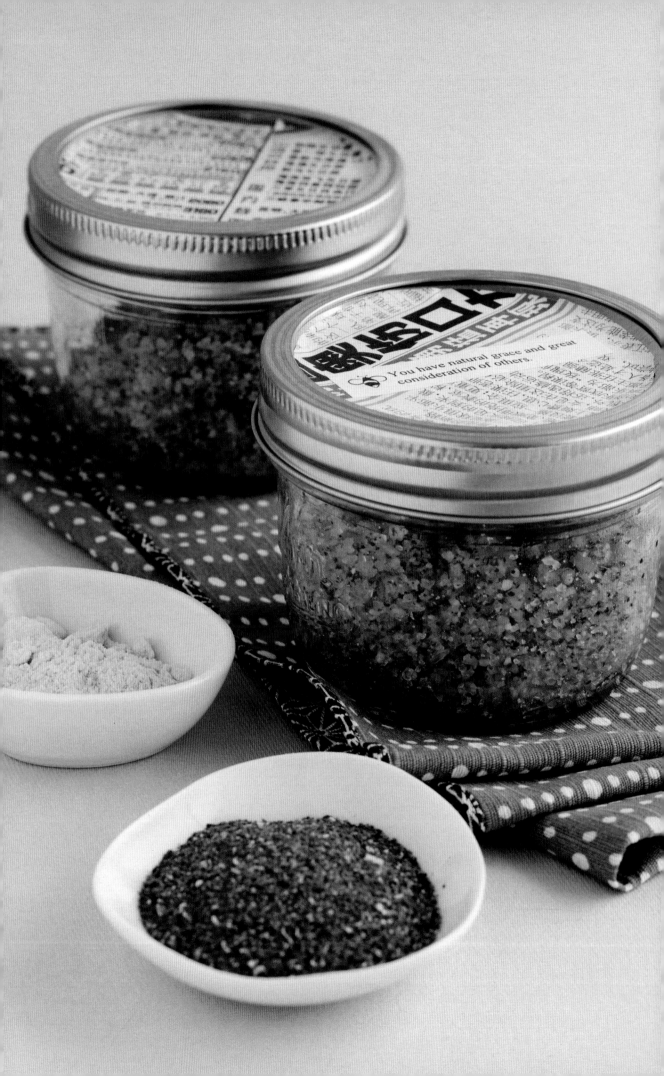

Sushi Body Scrub

Both my sister and I love sushi. When we want to catch up with each other, we always plan a special meal at our favorite sushi spot. But as you'll see in this recipe, sushi isn't just for eating anymore! In fact, many cosmetics companies now feature rice scrubs in their product lines because they're gentle and effective for getting skin really clean and smooth. Ground rice acts like a million tiny loofah sponges to polish your body. Use a clean coffee grinder or food processor to grind up the rice (and the seaweed, if need be).

1 cup ground uncooked rice
1 tablespoon powdered kelp
  or seaweed
¼ teaspoon wasabi powder
2 tablespoons light sesame oil
1 teaspoon rice vinegar

Stir all of the ingredients until well mixed. Spoon the scrub into a clean jar with a tight-fitting lid and store it in a cool, dry location, where it will keep for about 4 weeks.

To use, massage the scrub into damp skin in a circular motion, then rinse well with warm water.

Yield: 9 ounces

QUICK TIP: For an easy body polish, use an all-natural loofah sponge. Loofah sponges are actually plants that are related to gourds. If you want to exercise your green thumb, try growing your own in the garden. You can find the seeds at most garden stores. They're large and easy to plant, and in most areas they should produce loofahs in about seventy-five days.

Sweet as Sugar Skin Scrub

This is my go-to recipe whenever I feel like I need to slough off some dead skin. I quickly mix up some sugar and a light oil such as walnut oil, sweet almond oil, or light sesame oil. It's oh so simple, but very effective for creating healthy, glowing skin.

1 cup raw sugar

¼ cup walnut oil or another
   light oil

½ teaspoon vitamin E oil

Stir all the ingredients together until well mixed. Spoon the scrub into a clean jar with a tight-fitting lid and store it in a cool, dry location. It tends to separate, so you may need to give it a stir before each use.

To use, stand in the shower or tub and massage a tablespoon or two of the scrub all over your body to gently exfoliate and moisturize your skin. Rinse well afterward. If you feel you need more moisture, follow up with a light cream or natural oil.

Yield: 10 ounces

Spa-Style Salt Rub

If you like to read spa menus like I do, you've undoubtedly noticed that almost all of them offer some type of salt scrub, rub, or exfoliating treatment. Salt has been used throughout history to clean and deodorize the skin. This scrub is great for skin that needs some serious exfoliation. For extra scrubbing power, use a natural loofah sponge to apply the mixture. You can substitute other oils for the almond oil if you like; avocado oil, sunflower oil, and light olive oil all work well here. Choose your favorite scent, or use different scents for different effects, such as lavender for relaxation, peppermint for energy, or rosemary to boost memory.

2 cups kosher salt

1 cup almond oil

2 to 3 drops essential oil
   (optional)

Stir all of the ingredients together until you have a thick paste. Spoon the scrub into a clean jar with a tight-fitting lid and store it in a cool, dry location, where it will keep for 1 to 2 months.

To use, stand in the shower or tub, take a handful of the paste, and massage it into your skin, starting with your feet. Massage the paste all over your body. When you've finished and your body is covered, rinse well with warm water. Don't use soap, or you'll remove the oil and its moisturizing benefits.

Yield: 16 ounces

No More Cottage Cheese Thighs!

Caffeine is known as a great ingredient for promoting circulation and treating cellulite, which is why it's the main ingredient in many high-end cellulite treatments. This scrub combines powerful exfoliation with caffeine from the coffee grounds to help smooth your thighs and legs. The massage action is actually what does the most good in fighting cellulite, so make sure you use a vigorous circular motion. If you use this scrub regularly (in combination with exercise and a healthy diet), you should see improvements in a few weeks.

1 cup freshly ground coffee
¹/₂ cup brown sugar
¹/₂ cup sea salt
¹/₂ cup almond oil

Mix the coffee, sugar, and salt together, then pour in the almond oil and stir until well mixed. Spoon the scrub into a clean jar with a tight-fitting lid and store it in a cool, dry, dark spot, where it will keep for about 4 weeks.

To use, massage into clean skin in a circular motion, focusing on your upper thighs and back end where cellulite is most common. Massage your legs using strong, flowing strokes for at least 5 minutes to boost circulation.

Yield: 16 ounces

BEAUTY SMARTS: WHAT IS CELLULITE? Cellulite is actually very common and not something that affects only overweight individuals. It forms when fat cells beneath the skin enlarge, restricting blood flow and circulation and causing fluid buildup that further bloats the fat cells. This is often more a result of heredity than poor health habits. Because this unsightly condition often affects the rear end or thighs, it's sometimes referred to as cottage cheese thighs or orange peel legs. There isn't a miracle product that can rid your body of cellulite, so save your money. But the good news is, it can be smoothed out with massage and a healthy diet. If you exercise, massage the area with a good scrub twice a week, and avoid fatty and junk foods, you will see improvement.

Cooling Cucumber Body Mask

This cooling mask is ideal for soothing a bad sunburn. Fresh cucumber is refreshing and will draw the "heat" out of your skin. It can be a bit drying because cucumbers are naturally astringent, so after you use this body mask, follow up with a rich natural oil or body cream.

¼ cup boiling water

2 chamomile tea bags

1 whole cucumber with peel, chopped

¼ cup aloe vera gel

2 drops essential oil of lavender

Pour the boiling water over the tea bags to make a strong tea. Once the tea has cooled a bit, remove the tea bags, pressing them to extract as much tea as possible. Put the tea in a blender or food processor, add the cucumber, aloe vera, and lavender oil, and blend until you have a smooth mixture.

To use, spread the entire mixture over your body or the sunburned area using your fingers or a small paintbrush. Leave the mask on for 20 to 30 minutes. You may want to wrap up in an old sheet or large towel so you can sit down or lie down and relax. Afterward, rinse well with cool water, pat your skin dry, and don't forget to moisturize!

Yield: 4–5 ounces

SUPER SUNBURN SOOTHERS

One of the most important things you can do for your skin is to cover up with clothing or be sure to wear sunscreen. However, you may still get a sunburn despite your best intentions, and they can be very uncomfortable. Here are some natural ingredients that are very helpful for soothing a sunburn:

❋ Witch hazel

❋ Apple cider vinegar

❋ Cucumber juice

❋ Aloe vera gel

❋ Buttermilk

❋ Cornstarch*

❋ Baking soda*

Apply 1 to 2 cups of the soother of your choice using one of the following three methods, and be sure to use a good lotion or moisturizer afterward, as these cures can be drying:

1. Dip a thin fabric such as cheesecloth, silk, or cotton in the liquid, then wrap the cloth around your sunburned areas. You may have to repeat as the fabric dries.

2. Add 1 to 2 cups of the soother to your bathwater. Make sure the water is warm, not hot, since hot water will dry out sunburned skin.

3. Apply the soother directly to the affected area using a spray bottle. Don't rub the solution into your skin; let it dry and repeat if necessary.

* If using as soothing solution, mix 1 cup of water with 2 tablespoons of the powder.

Mixed Greens Body Mask

This is like a big green salad for your skin. It will get your body really clean and leave your skin well moisturized, soft, and smooth. Spinach and mushrooms are currently popular, if unexpected, body care ingredients that soothe, cleanse, and calm the skin.

2 cups loosely packed fresh spinach leaves

1/2 cup chopped mushrooms

1/2 cup loosely packed chopped parsley

1/2 fresh cucumber with peel, chopped

2 tablespoons white clay powder

1 tablespoon light olive oil, plus extra for moisturizing afterward

1 tablespoon apple cider vinegar

Combine all of the ingredients in a blender or food processor and blend until you have a smooth green paste.

To use, spread the entire mixture all over your body using your fingertips or a small paintbrush. Leave the mask on for 15 to 20 minutes. You may want to wrap up in an old sheet or large towel so you can sit down or lie down and relax. Afterward, rinse well with warm water, pat your skin dry, and massage some light olive oil into your skin.

Yield: 12 ounces

GREAT GIFT: GREEN BEAUTY

Start with a recycled basket or Easy Brown Paper Sack Basket (page 144) and put in a jar of Mixed Greens Body Mask (with a note to keep it refrigerated), along with some other green beauty products (preferably homemade!). Include a low-flow showerhead, organic cotton washcloths, and organic cotton balls and cotton swabs. Fill any remaining spaces with fresh fruits and vegetables. Everyone can use a little green in their beauty routine.

Oatmeal Cookie Bath

This is one of my favorite baths for unwinding before bed at the end of a long day, and it makes a fun gift for a friend. Simply pour the dry mixture into a jar and cover it with a bit of cotton fabric tied up with a ribbon, and maybe a cinnamon stick. Include a gift card with instructions for using the bath. For a real treat, you could also include some homemade oatmeal cookies and a good book. Oatmeal is very softening to the skin. Make sure to moisturize your skin very well after soaking in this bath.

1 cup rolled oats
¹/₂ cup baking soda
¹/₂ teaspoon ground cinnamon
1 tablespoon vanilla extract

Put all of the ingredients in a blender or food processor and blend on high speed until you have a smooth mixture like whole-grain flour.

To use, pour the entire mixture under running water while drawing a bath. Relax in the tub and enjoy!

Yield: 8 ounces

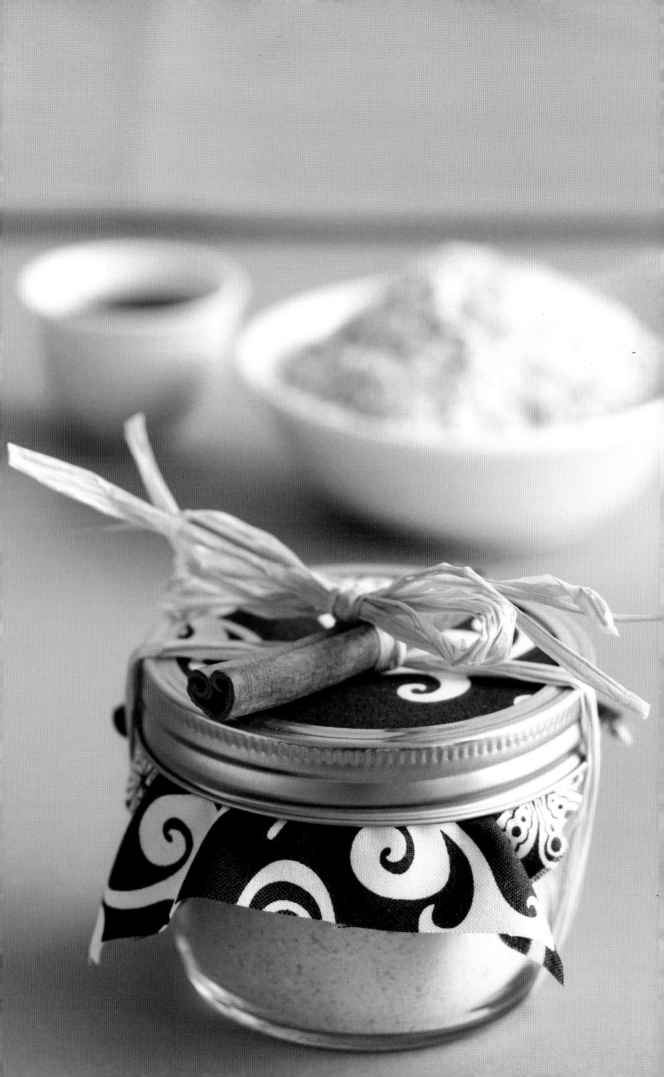

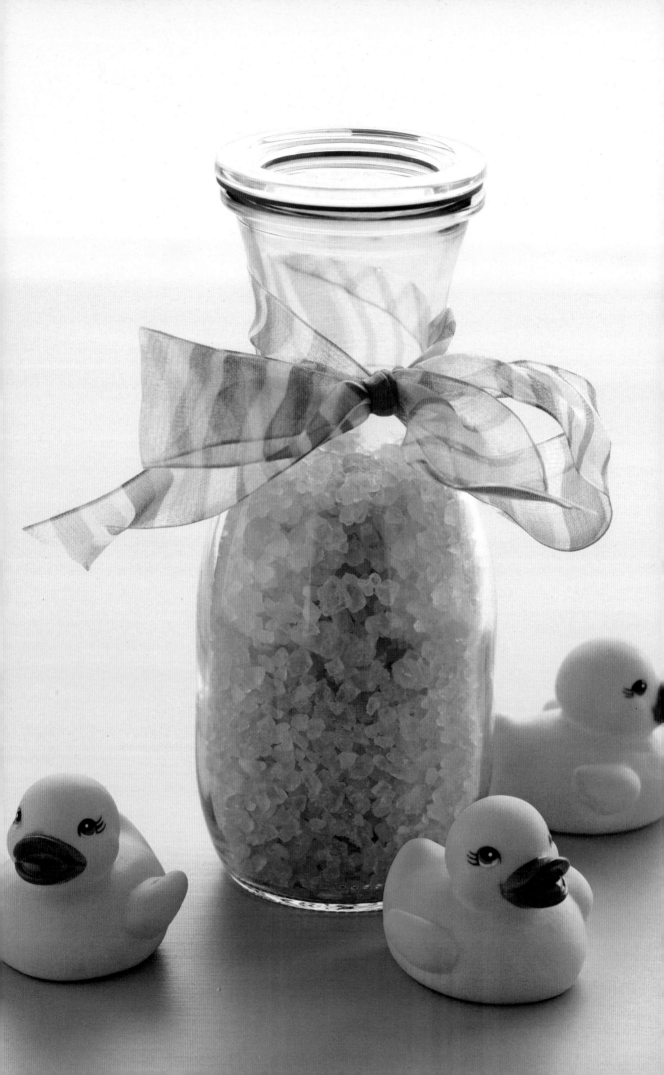

Bubbly Bath Salts

This recipe combines the fun of a bubble bath with the muscle-soothing power of bath salts. I love to give this to my friends as a gift, packaged in a fun container, along with a bright washcloth or rubber ducky.

$1/2$ **cup liquid soap**

1 tablespoon light oil, such as canola, sunflower, or almond

3 to 4 drops food coloring (optional)

6 cups rock salt or kosher salt

Stir the soap, oil, and food coloring together. Pour this mixture over the rock salt and stir until the salt crystals are evenly coated. Spread the salt out in a thin layer on a cookie sheet covered with wax paper and allow it to air-dry until all of the moisture has evaporated. This can take up to a full day; if you want to speed the process, put the salt in the oven on the lowest heat setting (without the wax paper).

To use, pour $1/4$ cup of the salts under running water while drawing a bath. Relax in the tub and enjoy!

Yield: 48 ounces

COLOR YOUR WORLD

Color is visible light energy and is used in bath and beauty products to enhance your senses or create a mood. Natural earth tones and pastel colors such as blue, green, and pink can be relaxing, while bold, vibrant colors such as orange, yellow, and red can be warming and energizing. When making your own products, you get to decide whether to add color or leave it out. You can use the food coloring found in the baking section of your grocery store (it may be synthetically produced, but I figure if it's safe to eat, then your skin won't mind a couple drops!). For all-natural choices, try exploring natural food stores and websites. Or if you're feeling adventurous, experiment with your own homemade colors using herbs, spices, and other natural ingredients from the list below.

Pink to Red: Beets, raspberries, red clay, hibiscus tea, paprika

Green: Liquid chlorophyll, green clay, spinach juice

Yellow: Turmeric, mustard powder

Orange: Carrot juice, calendula petals

Blue to Purple: Blueberries, red cabbage, lavender flowers

To extract the color from spices or flower petals, mix them with equal parts witch hazel or boiling water, let the mixture steep for several hours, then strain out any solids. Add the colored liquid to the recipe, a few drops at a time, until you create a shade you love!

Hot Cocoa Bath

Milk baths are great for the skin because the lactic acid in milk helps to smooth and soften skin. Chocolate milk is even better for your skin because it has all the softening powers of milk along with the antioxidant benefits of chocolate. This bath made with chocolate milk is a yummy treat to refresh your skin. You might even want to make a cup of hot chocolate to enjoy in the tub!

2 cups chocolate milk
2 tablespoons mild liquid
  soap, such as castile
1 tablespoon honey

Stir all of the ingredients together until well mixed.

To use, pour the entire mixture under running water while drawing a bath. Relax in the tub and enjoy!

Yield: 17 ounces

Hollywood Bubble Bath

If you want a Hollywood-style bubble bath, just like Julia Roberts in *Pretty Woman*, this is the recipe for you. It creates the perfect bubbly hideout at the end of a long day or the start of a new one. When I come home from college, I always treat myself to an entire day of pampering, and I always start by relaxing in this bubble bath and reading all of the old magazines my mom has saved for me.

1/2 cup mild liquid soap,
  such as castile
1 tablespoon sugar or honey
1 egg white

Stir all of the ingredients together until well mixed.

To use, pour the entire mixture under running water while drawing a bath. Relax in the tub and enjoy!

Yield: 6 ounces

ECO TIP: Recycle your soap scraps by grating them into flakes and placing them in small dishes next to your sink to use when your wash your hands and face. This also works well with small soaps from hotels, which are usually thrown out after just one use. You can also add soap flakes to bath salts, body scrubs, molded soaps, and foot soaks, or use them to make liquid soap (see page 6).

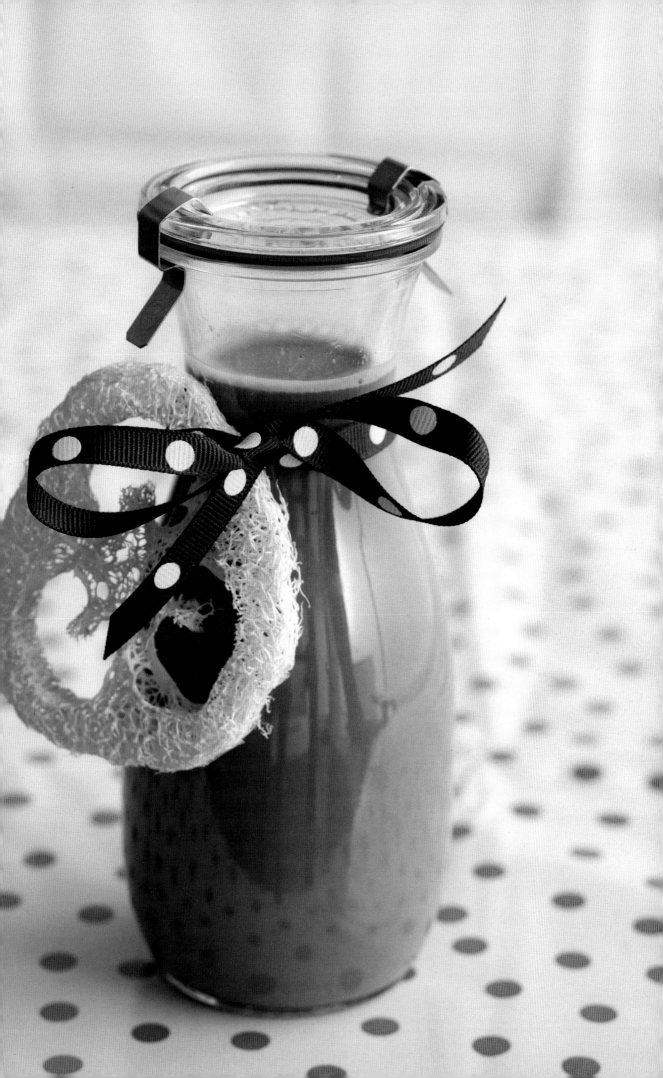

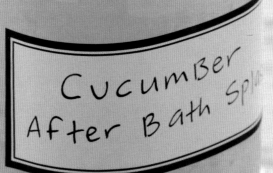

Cucumber
After Bath Spl...

Cucumber After-Bath Splash

After-bath splashes or sprays are meant to be used all over your body after a bath or shower to refresh your skin and close your pores, sort of like a toner for your whole body. Fresh cucumber juice and mint make this a refreshing splash with a clean, green scent. In the summer months I like to keep it in the fridge for a cool treat.

½ **fresh cucumber with peel,**
   chopped
½ **cup distilled water**
2 **tablespoons chopped**
   fresh mint leaves, or
   1 tablespoon dried

Put all of the ingredients in a blender or food processor and blend until smooth. Pour the mixture through a fine-mesh sieve to remove all of the solids, then pour into a clean spray bottle. Store it in the refrigerator, where it will keep 1 to 2 weeks.

To use, splash or spray on clean skin after bathing.

Yield: 4 ounces

QUICK TIP: The greatest skin toner of all is ice-cold water, so turn your shower tap to the coldest setting you can stand at the end of your shower. It will also energize your entire body!

Scented Shower Gels

Scented shower gels are so convenient to use, and it's easy to make them at home using your favorite scents or essential oils. This recipe is also a huge money saver—just buy unscented liquid soap by the gallon and transform it into your own unique blends. For containers, you can reuse plastic water bottles; the sport-style bottles with push/pull tops work really well for shower gels. They're the perfect size and won't break if dropped in the shower. Plus, if you keep a few bottles from hitting the landfill, this shower gel will make for a cleaner you *and* a cleaner planet.

½ cup unscented liquid soap
1 teaspoon light oil, such as canola, sunflower, or almond
4 to 5 drops essential oil

Stir all of the ingredients together until well mixed. Pour the shower gel into a clean plastic bottle with a push/pull top.

To use, pour a bit of shower gel into your hands and massage it into damp skin while you shower, or use a shower sponge. Rinse well afterward. You can also pour some under running water while drawing a bath for an instant scented bubble bath.

Yield: 4 ounces

ECO TIP: Reusing plastic drink bottles couldn't be easier. Simply wash them well, remove all of the labels, and let them air-dry. If you want to label homemade products you'll be using in the bath or shower, it's a good idea to label your bottle with a water-proof or permanent marker. Another way to reuse plastic bottles is to cut them in half to make two useful home beauty tools. The top half with the pour spout is a great funnel, and the bottom half can be used as a mold for homemade soaps and bath bombs.

SHOWER GEL SCENTS

Choose one or a combination of the following scents to create a specific mood:

Energizing	Calming	Romantic	Bold
Orange	Chamomile	Rose	Patchouli
Jasmine	Vanilla	Peach	Rosemary
Peppermint	Lavender	Cinnamon	Lemongrass
Cedar			

Deodorant Body Powder

I like to work out and go to the gym. The only downside is body odor—something you definitely don't want to have! I keep this simple powder in my gym bag and sprinkle it inside my running shoes because it helps neutralize odor-causing bacteria (sounds like a commercial, but hey, it's true!). You can also use it directly on your body. You can find liquid chlorophyll at most drugstores.

1 cup cornstarch
1 tablespoon baking soda
1 teaspoon liquid chlorophyll

Stir all of the ingredients together until well mixed. I like to do this in a large resealable plastic bag, as you can seal it and massage the mixture until the chlorophyll is thoroughly distributed. Pour the powder into a clean container, preferably one with a shaker top.

To use, sprinkle the powder on your skin, or place it in a small bowl and use a powder puff to powder your entire body.

Yield: 8 ounces

BEAUTY SMARTS: WHAT CAUSES BODY ODOR? You have millions of sweat glands, and when your body temperature heats up, you perspire, sweat, or, as my grandmother says, "glow." Fresh sweat or perspiration is made up of water, salt, and electrolytes and doesn't have a scent. However, when it remains on your skin, bacteria begin to break it down, and this is what causes body odor. There are many factors that affect how much you sweat, including heredity, diet, medication, and, for women, the time of the month. Keeping your skin clean, dry, and healthy should help control body odor. I use a simple body powder of cornstarch and baking soda to help keep my body smelling good.

Moisturizing Body Powder

I like to use this body powder in the winter months, when my skin needs all the extra moisture it can get. I like the sweet scent of vanilla, but you can substitute your favorite essential oil in this recipe, or even a favorite perfume or cologne.

½ **cup rice flour**
½ **cup cornstarch**
½ **teaspoon almond oil**
½ **teaspoon vanilla extract**

Stir all of the ingredients together until well mixed. I like to do this in a large resealable plastic bag, as you can seal it and massage the mixture until the oil and scent are thoroughly distributed. Pour the powder into a clean container, preferably one with a shaker top.

To use, sprinkle the powder on your skin, or place it in a small bowl and use a powder puff to powder your entire body.

Yield: 8 ounces

SIMPLE SCENTED POWDERS

Cornstarch has been used as a body powder for ages. It's one of the first things I learned from my great-grandmother, who also used to sprinkle scented powder onto her sheets before bed each night. For a super simple scented body powder, simply place a cup of cornstarch in a resealable plastic bag and add a few drops of essential oil. Seal the bag and massage the contents until the scent is evenly distributed.

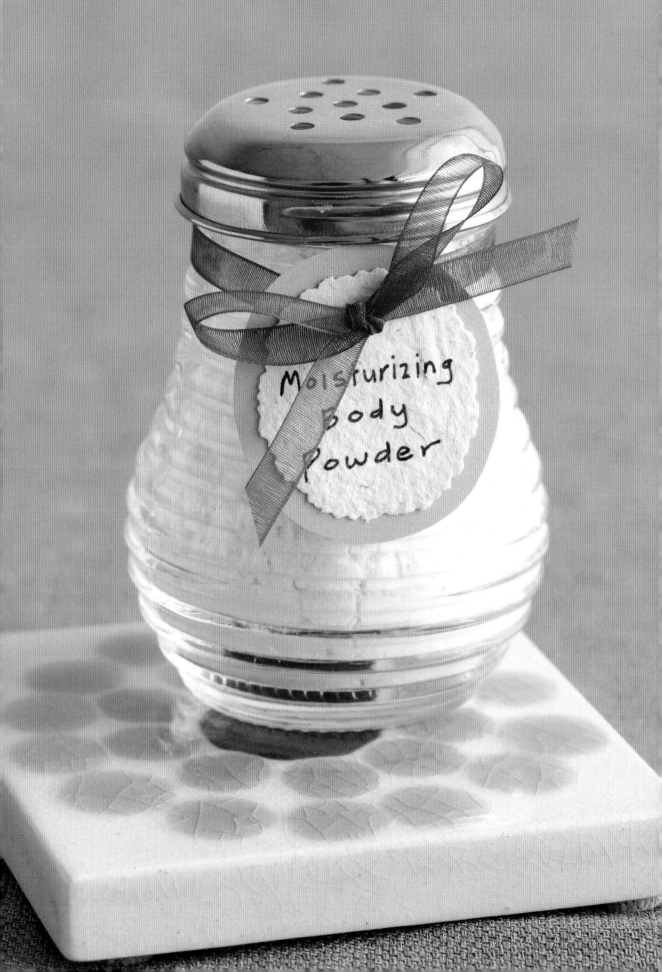

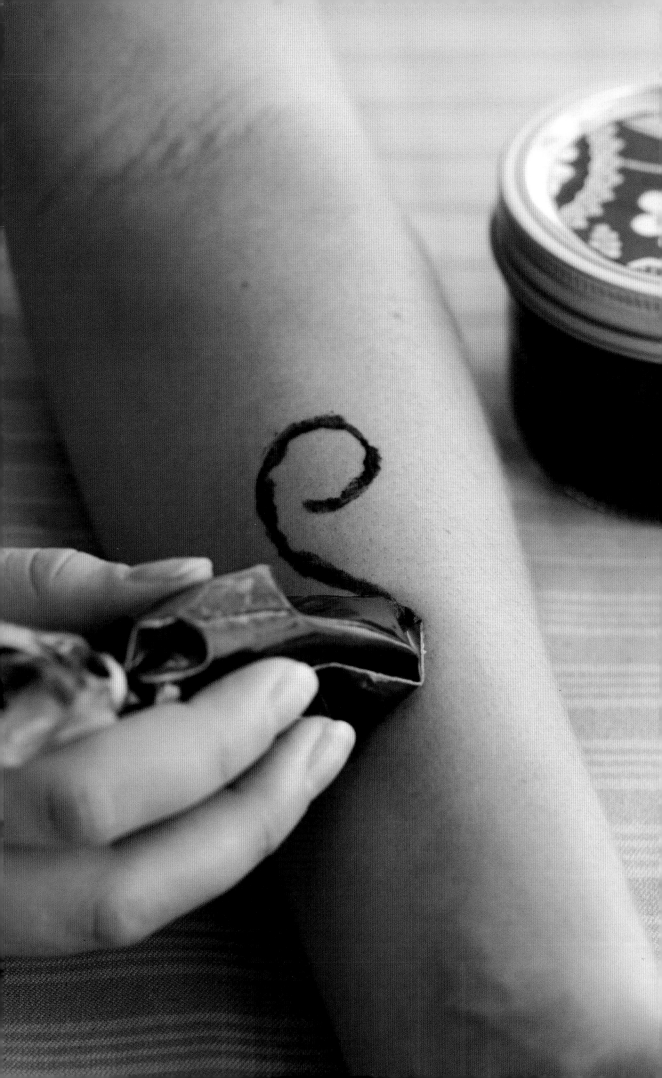

Henna Tattoos

When my sister and I were in Egypt, we discovered an all-natural and temporary type of body marking using henna, a practice known as mehndi. My sister and I both got tiny sun designs on our backs. It was fun, and best of all, they faded away when we were tired of them. You can find henna tattoo kits in many salons and craft stores, but it's just as easy to create your own using henna from a natural food store or drugstore. I recommend starting with a small, simple design such as a heart or dots and lines.

¹/₄ cup boiling water
2 tea bags (orange pekoe
    or black tea works best)
¹/₄ cup henna powder,
    finely sifted
Lemon slices

Pour the boiling water over the tea bags, let it steep for at least 1 hour, then remove the tea bags, pressing them to extract as much tea as possible. Place the sifted henna in a glass or ceramic bowl, then slowly add the tea, stirring continuously until you have a smooth, creamy paste; you may not need to use all of the tea. Let the mixture sit for several hours or even overnight to extract as much color as possible from the henna. If the mixture seems too dry, add a bit more water or tea and stir well. It should have the consistency of toothpaste and be easy to spread. Decide on your design and where you want it to go. Before applying the henna, wash the area with a mild soap cleanser, then pat your skin dry (lotions and even the skin's natural oils can prevent the henna from working).

To paint with your henna paste, place it in a pastry bag or a plastic bag with one corner snipped off, or use a small brush. Apply the henna carefully, since it will stain. Once you've finished your design, let the henna dry on your skin, dabbing it every now and then with a slice of lemon; the acidity of the lemon juice will help set the design, and the moisture will help the dye slowly absorb into the skin. Some people leave the henna on overnight for a darker color. I've let mine sit for just a few hours and was satisfied with the color.

When you're ready, rinse off the henna with warm water and rub the design with more lemon juice. Voilà! Your design will darken a bit more as the lemon juice dries. Your tattoo should last for several weeks, depending upon where it is and how often you wash it.

Yield: 2 ounces

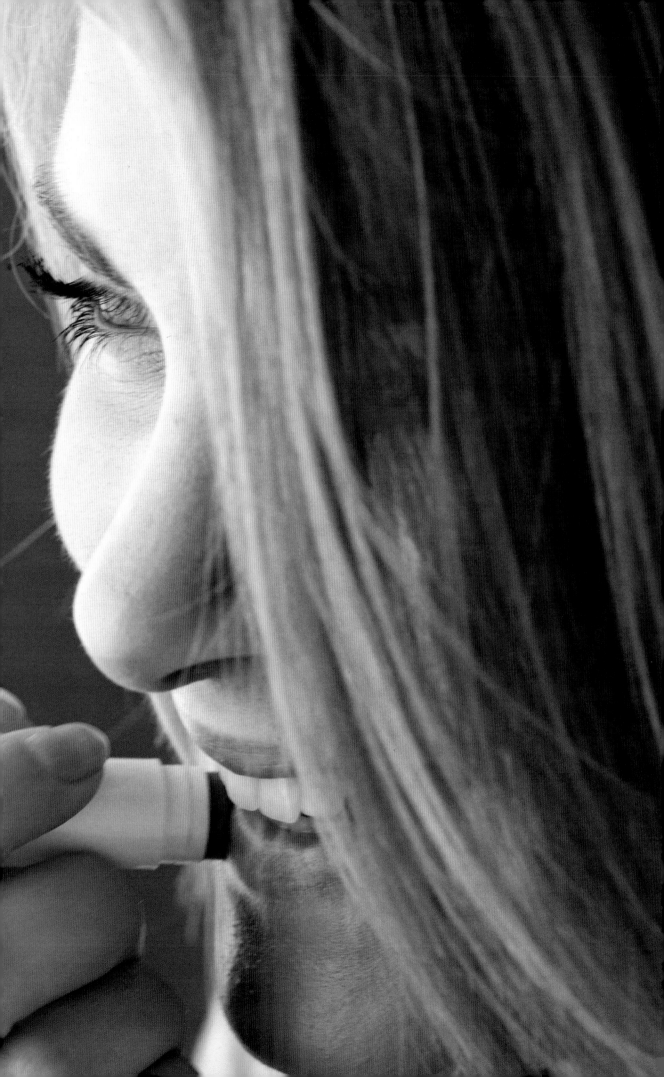

FOR THE MOUTH

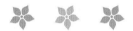

Have you ever noticed that on all of those makeover shows they always focus on the person's mouth? They give them a new smile or a bright new lip color and it makes a huge difference.

Your mouth is a focal point of your face, and a great smile makes all the difference in how you look and feel. When you smile, the world smiles with you! Your mouth is also the center of some pretty important activities, such as eating, drinking, breathing, talking, and kissing. So taking good care of your mouth, teeth, and lips is important, and it's actually pretty easy to achieve.

The two most important aspects of mouth care are also the most obvious: brushing and flossing to help rid your mouth of bacteria and keep it fresh and clean. Nothing is worse than bad breath. We all know people who are fun to be around but have stinky breath and no one wants to tell them. You may wonder why they don't notice it themselves, but it's probably because we get used to our own bad breath, and if no one ever tells us about it, then we never know! So do these people a favor and hand them a sprig of parsley or breath mint. Hopefully, you'll get a little fresh breath karma and someone will do the same for you.

Dry conditions and environments actually make bad breath worse, because saliva cleanses the mouth. This is why our breath is usually worse in the morning. Make sure you keep your mouth moist by drinking plenty of water and water-based beverages. Coffee and black tea aren't helpful, since they're naturally dehydrating. Plus, they can stain your teeth. Also, try to cut down on the amount of soda and other acidic drinks you consume, since they're hard on tooth enamel.

Besides your teeth and gums, it's important to take care of your lips. The lips are one of the most sensitive areas of the body. They also get a lot of exposure to harsh weather conditions, such as sun, wind, and excessive cold, so it's important to protect them with lip balms and conditioners. I like simple mixtures that are rich in natural oils and vegetable fats, such as coconut oil or cocoa butter. It's also a good idea to gently exfoliate your lips with a soft toothbrush or cotton washcloth from time to time. I usually scrub my lips once a week to keep them looking their best. If you suffer from chapped or extremely dry lips you may need to do this more often. Use the recipes in this chapter to take good care of your teeth, mouth, and lips, and don't forget to *smile*. Not only will it enhance your appearance, it's also good for your overall well-being and outlook on life—and it will make the people around you feel better too!

NATURAL MOUTH FRESHENERS

There are several natural mouth fresheners you can nibble on after a meal or anytime your breath needs freshening. Be sure to rinse well afterwards to cleanse any bits of spice or herbs from your teeth.

❋ Anise seeds

❋ Clove buds

❋ Fennel seeds

❋ Gingerroot

❋ Mint leaves

❋ Parsley sprigs

❋ Strawberry hulls
(the small green cap
on fresh strawberries)

TEN TIPS FOR A HAPPY MOUTH

A fresh, clean mouth is a happy mouth, so here are ten simple things you can do to keep your mouth, lips, and teeth healthy and looking their best:

1. Flossing is the most important thing you can do for healthy teeth and gums; try to do it twice a day.

2. Brush your teeth twice a day.

3. For strong, healthy teeth, make sure you have enough calcium and vitamins C and D in your diet.

4. Boost circulation and exfoliate dead skin by brushing your lips with a soft toothbrush.

5. Protect your lips with a rich lip balm or natural oil such as coconut oil.

6. Avoid licking your lips, which will actually dry them out.

7. After drinking colas, coffee, or tea, which can stain your teeth, drink a glass of water.

8. Brush your tongue to help combat bad breath.

9. Keep your mouth well hydrated by drinking plenty of water.

10. Smile! And don't forget to visit your dentist every year.

Major Moisture Lip Balm

Packed with moisturizing agents, this lip balm is the answer for dry lips! Whenever my lips are dry or chapped, especially during the winter months, this is what I automatically reach for. It also makes a great gift or stocking stuffer around the holiday season. Just add a seasonal ribbon or a holiday-themed label and you're set!

1 teaspoon coconut or palm oil
$\frac{1}{2}$ teaspoon castor oil
$\frac{1}{2}$ teaspoon grated beeswax
$\frac{1}{2}$ teaspoon almond oil
$\frac{1}{8}$ teaspoon vitamin E oil

Put all of the ingredients in a small microwave-safe container and microwave on low heat for 1 to 2 minutes, just until the beeswax has melted. (You could also do this on the stovetop, preferably in a double boiler. Since it's kind of a pain using a saucepan with such small amounts of ingredients, you might want to make multiple batches at once. To make a smaller batch on the stovetop, place a glass measuring cup inside a pan filled with a few inches of water.) Stir the mixture until everything is evenly combined, then allow it to cool completely. Once it's cool, spoon the lip balm into a small, clean container.

To use, spread the lip balm on your lips and enjoy!

Yield: $\frac{1}{2}$ ounce

CHAPPED LIP CURE

Here's a simple cure for painfully chapped lips: Mix together equal parts of lemon juice and castor oil. Before you go to bed, spread the mixture over your lips and leave it on overnight. You'll wake up to smooth and soothed lips. And, of course, use a rich lip balm on your lips during the day.

Luscious Lips Balm

This basic lip balm is super simple to make, and you can wear it under or over a lip color for extra shine and conditioning. Coconut oil is a great lip conditioner, creating a protective layer on your lips that really locks in moisture. You can find it in the grocery store or at Asian markets. If you want to spice up this recipe, add a bit of essential oil or flavoring extract. Citrus is my favorite in this recipe.

1 teaspoon coconut oil
1 teaspoon almond oil
1/2 teaspoon grated beeswax

Put all of the ingredients in a small microwave-safe container and microwave on low heat for 1 to 2 minutes, until the beeswax has melted. (You could also do this on the stovetop, preferably in a double boiler. Since it's kind of a pain using a saucepan with such small amounts of ingredients, you might want to make multiple batches at once. To make a smaller batch on the stovetop, place a glass measuring cup inside a pan filled with a few inches of water.) Stir until all of the ingredients are well mixed, then pour the mixture into a small, clean container and let it cool completely.

To use, spread the lip balm on your lips and enjoy!

Yield: 1/2 ounce

QUICK TIP: Recycle old lipstick tubes and small jars to hold your homemade lip balms. This is easy to do: simply remove as much of the old lipstick or lip balm as you can with a small knife, then soak the tube in very hot water. Allow it to air-dry, or roll up a bit of paper towel and insert into the tube to absorb any leftover moisture.

Very Vanilla Lip Gloss

My favorite flower is the orchid and vanilla comes from a type of orchid native to Mexico, so it just makes sense that this is my favorite lip gloss recipe. It's easy to make and tastes just like a vanilla ice cream cone. I like to use organic vanilla extract in this recipe; it smells so good that sometimes I even dab it behind my ears and on my wrists as a perfume. You can also use vanilla-flavored oil, which you can find at gourmet cooking stores, for the flavoring. The coconut oil and vitamin E oil will keep your lips conditioned and soft.

1 teaspoon grated beeswax
1 teaspoon coconut oil
1/8 teaspoon vitamin E oil
1/8 teaspoon pure vanilla
    extract or vanilla-
    flavored oil

Put the beeswax, coconut oil, and vitamin E oil in a small microwave-safe container and microwave on low heat for 1 to 2 minutes, until the beeswax has melted. (You could also do this on the stovetop, preferably in a double boiler. Since it's kind of a pain using a saucepan with such small amounts of ingredients, you might want to make multiple batches at once. To make a smaller batch on the stovetop, place a glass measuring cup inside a pan filled with a few inches of water.) Add the vanilla extract and stir until well mixed. Pour the mixture into a small, clean container and let it cool completely.

To use, spread the gloss onto your lips and enjoy!

Yield: 1/2 ounce

BEAUTY SMARTS: WHAT'S THE HISTORY OF LIPSTICK?

Lip products go way back in history. Lip paints were used in Mesopotamia as early as 3500 BCE, and in early New England prim Puritan women whipped up lip balm using crushed rose petals. In 1910, lipstick as we know it today was invented in Paris. It is now the most commonly used and purchased cosmetic product in the world, and no wonder—I know I can always use a new lip balm!

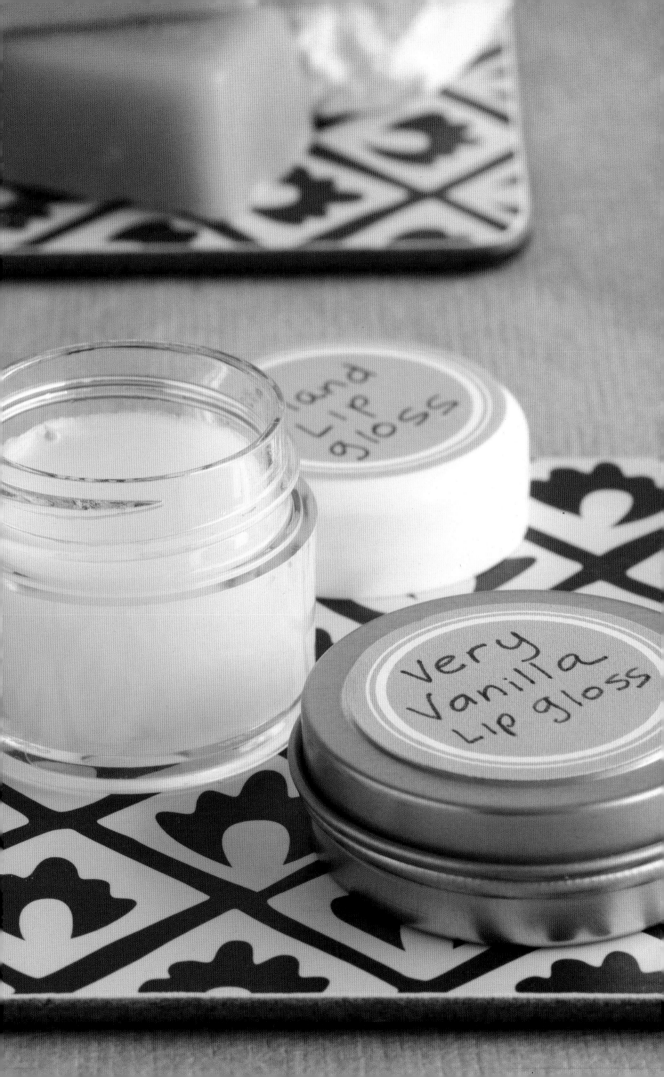

Island Lip Gloss

Made with natural oils straight from the islands, this lip gloss is full of moisture and feels like taking a trip to the tropics. Slick this on in the cold winter months when you could use a vacation to Hawaii and your lips could use the moisture. If you can't find macadamia nut oil, you can substitute any light oil, such as almond, walnut, or light sesame oil.

1 teaspoon grated beeswax

1 teaspoon grated cocoa butter

1 teaspoon coconut oil

1 teaspoon macadamia nut oil

1 teaspoon light sesame oil

1/8 teaspoon vitamin E oil

Put all of the ingredients in a small microwave-safe container and microwave on low heat for 1 to 2 minutes, just until the beeswax has melted. (You could also do this on the stovetop, preferably in a double boiler. Since it's kind of a pain using a saucepan with such small amounts of ingredients, you might want to make multiple batches at once. To make a smaller batch on the stovetop, place a glass measuring cup inside a pan filled with a few inches of water.) Stir until all of the ingredients are well mixed, then pour the mixture into a small, clean container.

To use, spread the gloss onto your lips and enjoy!

Yield: 3/4 ounce

Lip Exfoliator

When it comes to exfoliating, the lips are often neglected. However, they can use exfoliation just as much as the rest of the body. This scrub will help you solve chapped lips or avoid them altogether. Just make sure to be very gentle when exfoliating your lips, as the skin is very delicate.

1 teaspoon almond oil

1 teaspoon honey

2 teaspoons brown sugar

Stir all of the ingredients together until you have a smooth paste. If you have any leftover mixture, store it in a small container in a dry, dark spot.

To use, gently massage a bit of the mixture into your lips using your fingertips. Rinse well with warm water, then enjoy your softer lips!

Yield: 1/2 ounce

Chocolate Brownie Lip Gloss

I love to bake for my friends, and rich chocolate brownies are one of my favorite things to make. This lip gloss is also a favorite recipe because it smells just like brownies and has the same great taste, but without the calories. It's extremely moisturizing and will keep your lips soft and kissable—and tasty!

1 tablespoon grated cocoa
  butter
1½ tablespoons coconut oil
2 teaspoons grated beeswax
½ teaspoon vitamin E oil
10 chocolate chips or
  1 teaspoon chopped
  chocolate

Combine all of the ingredients in a small microwave-safe container and microwave on low heat for about 1 minute, until melted. (You could also do this on the stovetop, preferably in a double boiler. Since it's kind of a pain using a saucepan with such small amounts of ingredients, you might want to make multiple batches at once. To make a smaller batch on the stovetop, place a glass measuring cup inside a pan filled with a few inches of water.) Stir until all of the ingredients are well mixed, then pour into small, clean containers. Allow the lip gloss to cool before using. (You can speed the process up by placing it in the refrigerator.)

To use, spread the gloss on your lips and enjoy!

Yield: 2 ounces

QUICK TIP: For an easy gourmet twist to this recipe, try adding 1 to 2 drops of flavored oil to the melted chocolate, such as raspberry, orange, cherry, peppermint, or coconut.

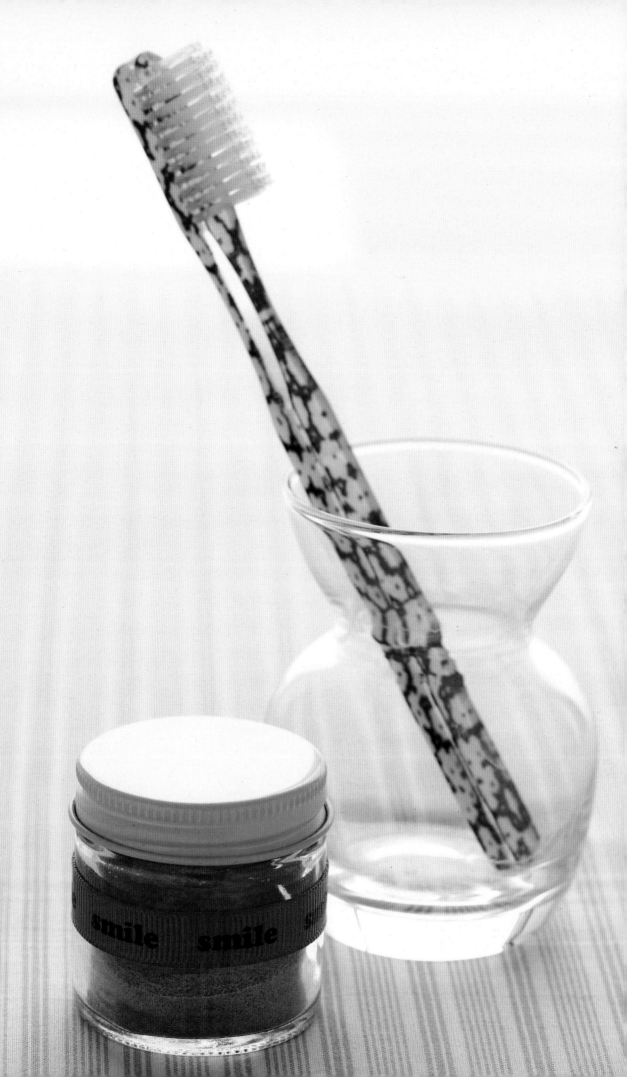

Cinnamon Toothpaste

Baking soda makes a great natural tooth powder. In this recipe, it's combined with cinnamon, which is a popular ingredient in toothpastes and mouthwashes because it helps kill the bacteria that cause tooth decay and gum disease. It also has a naturally sweet, spicy flavor that helps cover up the salty taste of the baking soda. This is a great natural alternative to store-bought toothpaste.

2 teaspoons baking soda
1 teaspoon ground cinnamon
2 teaspoons water

This recipe makes enough for a few uses, so mix it up in a small container with a tight-fitting lid. Simply put all of the ingredients in the container, then use the back of a spoon to stir until you have a smooth paste.

To use, spread a small amount of toothpaste onto a clean toothbrush and brush your teeth for 2 minutes, then rinse well.

Yield: ³/₄ ounce

Minty Toothpaste

Mint is the classic toothpaste flavor. This pale-colored gel is nonabrasive and gentle, making it a good choice for sensitive teeth and gums. I used it when I first got my braces and my mouth was adjusting to all of the new hardware on my teeth.

1 tablespoon chopped
  fresh mint leaves or
  ¹/₂ tablespoon dried
¹/₄ cup boiling water
¹/₂ teaspoon almond oil
¹/₂ teaspoon cornstarch

Put the mint leaves in a small glass bowl, pour in the boiling water, and let the mint steep as the water cools completely. Strain into a small microwave-safe container or small saucepan, then stir in the almond oil and cornstarch. Bring the mixture to a boil in the microwave or on the stovetop, then allow it to cool completely. Stir until all of the ingredients are well mixed, then spoon the gel into a small, clean container with a tight-fitting lid.

To use, spread a small amount of the gel on a clean toothbrush and brush your teeth for 2 minutes, then rinse well.

Yield: 2 ounces

Apple Juice Mouth Rinse

We all know that an apple a day can keep the doctor away, but did you know that they're also useful for keeping bad breath at bay? This refreshing and sweet mouth rinse also has antiseptic properties because of the fresh mint and ginger.

1/2 cup apple juice
1 tablespoon rose water
1 slice of fresh gingerroot
1 sprig of fresh mint

Put all of the ingredients in a clean container with a tight-fitting lid and shake gently to mix. Store this mouth rinse in the refrigerator between uses. It will keep for about 2 weeks.

To use, rinse your mouth with 1 or 2 teaspoons of the rinse for 30 seconds.

Yield: 4½ ounces

QUICK TIP: My mom always made me gargle with salt water if I had a sore throat. It also works wonders for sore gums and really kills all the bacteria in your mouth!

Simple Clove Mouthwash

Simply chewing on a clove bud will disinfect and freshen your breath. I keep a small tin of them in my purse for this purpose. Another way to use cloves is in this mouthwash, which is super simple to make and will help combat halitosis, or bad breath. Keep it in a pretty bottle next to your sink.

2 tablespoons whole cloves
2 cups boiling water

Place the cloves in a heat-resistant container, then pour in the boiling water. Cover the container and let the mixture sit until it's cool. Strain the mouthwash and pour it into a clean container.

To use, rinse your mouth with 1 teaspoon of the mouthwash for 30 seconds.

Yield: 16 ounces

ECO TIP: Turning off your faucet while you brush your teeth can save up to eight gallons of water per day.

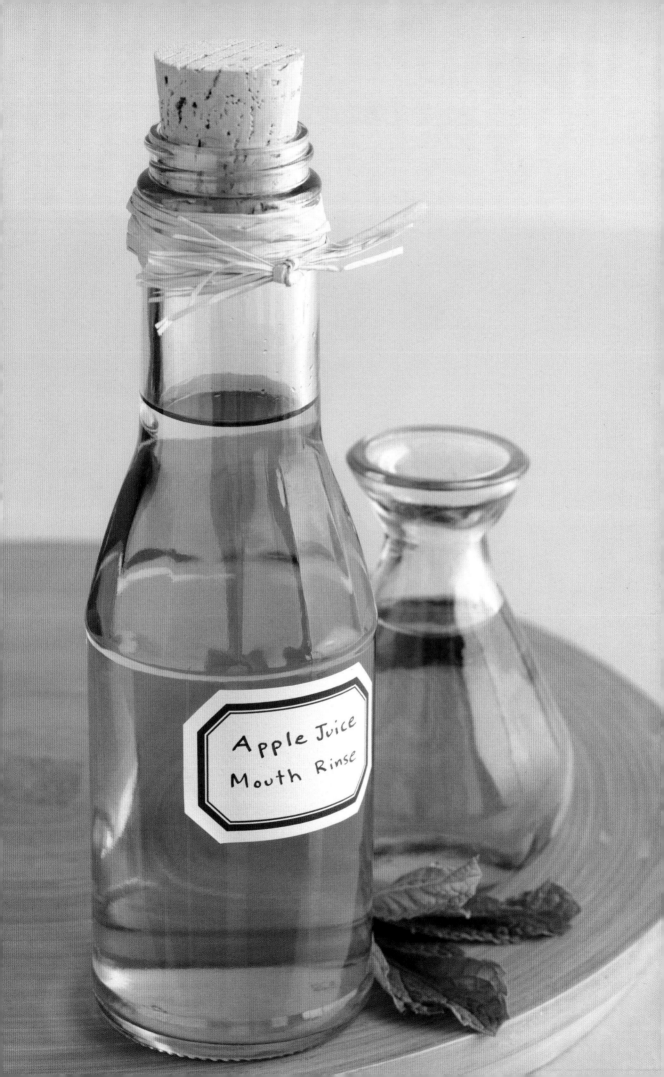

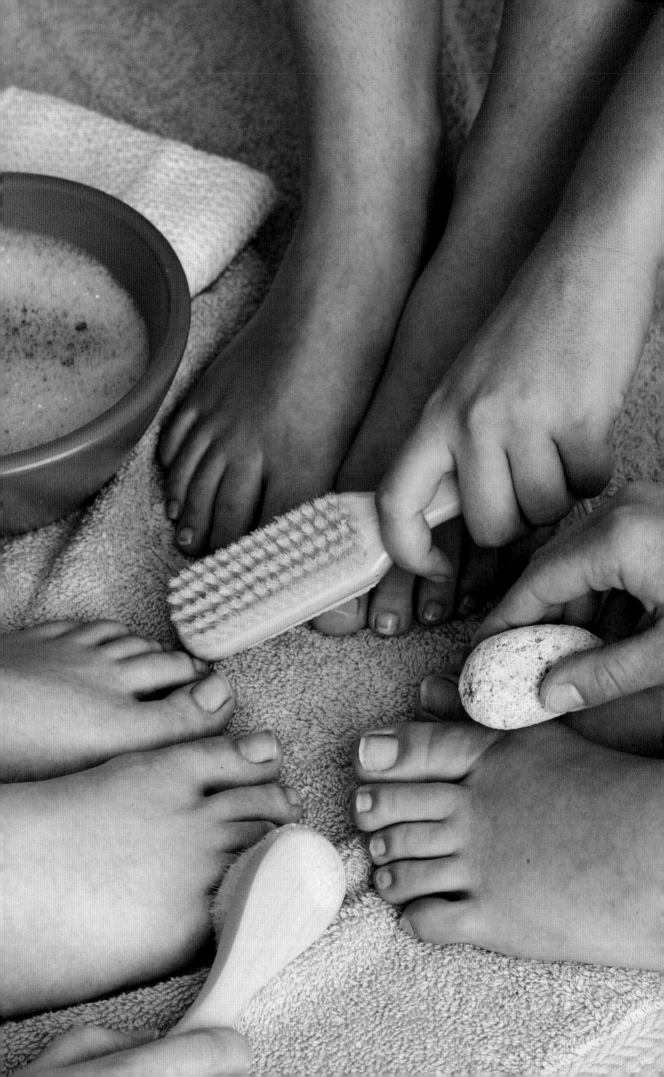

FOR THE HANDS AND FEET

It's easy to have healthy and attractive hands, feet, and nails. You don't have to book expensive manicures and pedicures or use a bunch of posh creams and nail oils. Just a few simple things, like keeping your nails well hydrated, will make a huge difference in how they look. Your hands need moisture more than any other part of your body because they have very few oil glands.

Nails are also very porous, which is another reason why it's important to keep them full of moisture. Apply nail creams and oils often to help lock in moisture. This is especially important after washing your hands, which the average person does at least five times a day. My mom keeps a bottle of lotion next to all the sinks in our house and encourages all of us to use it after washing our hands. I also keep a small bottle of hand cream in my purse. Massaging in a good cream or lotion will also boost circulation and help your nails grow.

It's important to protect your hands and nails when you do household chores or craft projects or anytime you work with harsh chemicals and toxic products that could damage or dry out your hands. Buy a pack of rubber gloves, and then be sure to use them. If you live in a cold climate, it also helps to wear gloves and mittens during the winter months, as extremely cold weather can be drying and hard on your skin.

Your hands are probably the hardest-working part of your body. They're involved in almost everything you do, from typing to working out. Your nails really do reflect your overall health, and a diet that's lacking in proper nutrients will show up as weak or flaking nails. For strong,

HOME SPA PARTY

Spas are nice places to go to relax and focus on yourself, but they're also pretty spendy. Why not plan a spa party instead? It's a great theme for a get-together, and a nice way to reconnect with and pamper your friends. I like to plan a spa party before a big dance or school event, when everyone wants to look and feel their best.

Your spa party can be a formal affair with invitations and planned activities, or a spontaneous, casual gathering when you notice people seem to be a bit bored or could use some cheering up. Here's how to set the mood for a spa party:

✽ **Sound:** Many spas play new age music or nature sounds. Burn a few CDs with relaxing tunes that will calm you down—or energize you if that's what you're looking for. Sometimes you need those sing-along girl power songs!

✽ **Color:** Believe it or not, color can have a big impact on your mood. For your spa party, choose calming natural colors such as blues, pinks, or greens for everything from towels and dishes to candles and flowers.

✽ **Refreshments:** Make up some special spa-style water by filling a glass pitcher with plenty of ice water and adding sliced cucumbers, mint leaves, or fresh berries. Also, have healthy, easy-to-eat treats on hand, and be sure they're made from fresh, all-natural ingredients. Fresh fruits and vegetables, hummus, and sushi all fit the bill. No junk food, please!

✽ **Spa activities:** Choose treatments that can easily be done in a group, such as manicures, pedicures, henna tattoos, and facial masks. You could also include other activities, like a nature stroll or a yoga session.

healthy nails, you need to eat a balanced diet with plenty of calcium and high-quality protein.

Never cut your cuticles. I know some people do this because they think it looks better, but it can cause hangnails, which are very painful. Also, your cuticles are meant to protect your nail bed from bacteria and infection, so you don't want to damage them. A better bet is to gently push them back, which is easier to do when they're wet. A simple habit to get into is to gently push back them back with a wet washcloth when you're showering or bathing.

Proper foot care is important year-round, not just during the summer months when you're wearing sandals and flip-flops. A good, simple pedicure weekly will do wonders for the health of your feet. It can also enhance your overall well-being if you add a little reflexology. Reflexology is the theory that different zones on the feet are related to different parts of the body, and that by massaging, squeezing, and pushing different areas of the feet you can improve your general health. I believe in this concept. I love a good foot massage, and it definitely gives me more energy!

Footbaths are another great way to treat your feet. You can use them as part of a pedicure, or anytime you want to revive and refresh your feet and remove rough skin. If you're involved in sports, a good foot soak is a great way to treat foot odor and revive tired muscles. You don't have to have a perfect mani/pedi all the time, but well-cared-for hands and feet do make a difference in how you feel.

TEN TIPS FOR STRONG HANDS AND SWEET FEET

Get ready to clap your hands and dance the night away—here are ten simple tips for healthy hands and feet that will keep them looking and feeling their best:

1. Keep your nails all the same length, shaped into square ovals, and well hydrated.

2. Give yourself a weekly manicure, and if you wear polish, let your nails breathe for one day each week.

3. Your nails are not tools! Don't use them to scrape, pick, pry, or scratch things.

4. Massage your nails daily to boost circulation and promote nail growth.

5. Never cut your cuticles.

6. Wear gloves when cleaning, working with chemicals, or painting.

7. Treat rough heels and feet with a pumice stone or foot scrub.

8. Give yourself a weekly pedicure to keep your feet healthy, even in the winter months when your feet are covered by boots and shoes and you think no one sees them!

9. After working out or playing sports, let your feet breathe and wear all natural cotton socks.

10. Eat a healthy, well-balanced diet with plenty of calcium and good-quality protein.

Lemon Sugar Hand Scrub

One of my passions is golfing. Whenever springtime rolls around, my hands start to get noticeably rougher from gripping the club. This scrub does a great job at defeating the calluses and rough areas on my hands and keeping them soft.

$1/2$ **cup sugar**
$1/2$ **cup Epsom salts**
6 drops lemon essential oil
3 tablespoons almond oil

Stir the sugar, Epsom salts, lemon essential oil, and almond oil together until well mixed. Pour the mixture into a clean container with a tight-fitting lid.

To use, first wash your hands, then massage a teaspoon or two of the hand scrub all over your hands. Rinse well with warm water and pat your hands dry.

Yield: 8 ounces

Red Grape Nail Scrub

Grapes are full of natural fruit acids. The red ones contain more antioxidants than the green ones, but both varieties will work in this recipe. The grape juice combined with sugar helps remove dead skin around your nails, eliminate hangnails, and condition your cuticles. This is a great treatment to do between manicures to keep your hands and nails looking their best. Afterward, keep the theme going with a grape seed oil hand massage.

10 red grapes, roughly
   chopped
2 tablespoons granulated
   sugar
Grape seed oil (optional)

Mix the grapes and sugar together using the back of a fork or small food processor. The mixture will be coarse in texture.

To use, massage a small amount of the nail scrub into the skin around each nail. Wipe off any excess, then massage a small amount of grape seed oil into your hands and nails.

Yield: 1 ounce

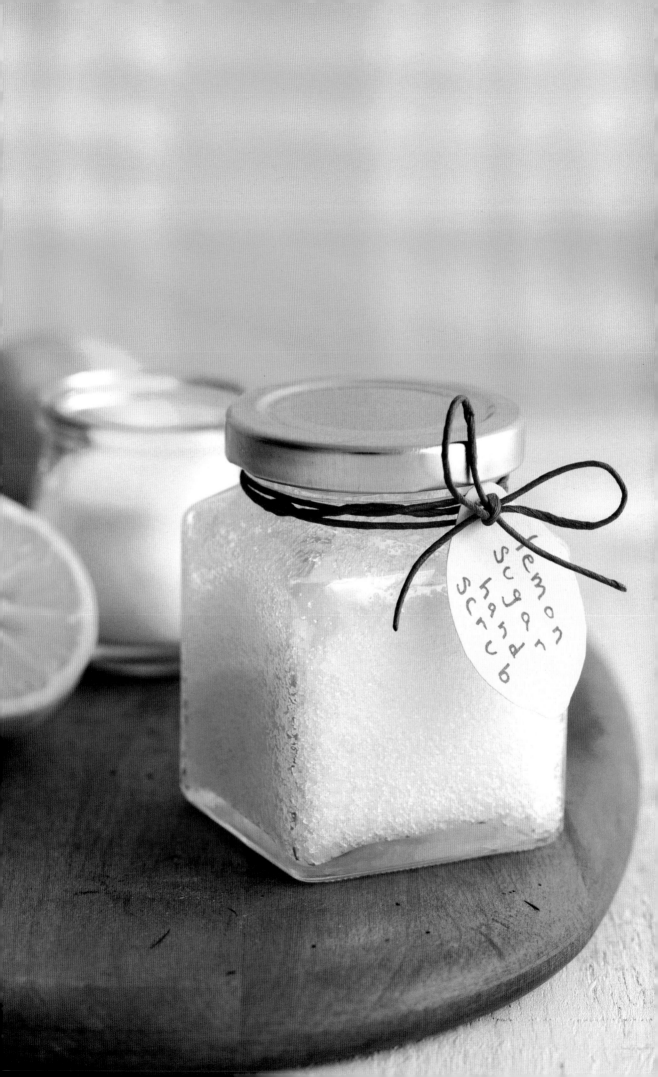

Marie's Basic Hand Cream

My sister Marie loves to make creams and lotions—in fact, she may be better at it than me! Her favorite thing to make is a basic hand cream that can be used all over, especially on classic rough skin spots such as elbows, knees, and heels. I think it is a bit too heavy for use on your face, but Marie disagrees and sometimes uses it as a night cream when her skin is really dry. It has a mild honey scent from the beeswax, but you may also add a drop or two of essential oils if you prefer a scented cream. We use natural borax powder from the grocery store in the laundry detergent aisle.

1/4 cup water
1/8 teaspoon borax powder
1/2 cup sunflower oil
2 tablespoons grated
   beeswax

Bring the water to a boil. Place the borax powder in a clean, heatproof bowl, pour in the boiling water, and stir well. Set aside. Place the oil and beeswax in a microwave-safe container, mix together, and microwave on high heat for 2 minutes, until the beeswax is melted. Pour the oil mixture into a blender or food processor and blend on low speed, adding the hot water mixture in a slow, steady stream. Blend on high speed until well mixed. Pour the mixture into a clean container to cool. You should have a white fluffy cream.

To use, massage into your skin.

Yield: 4 ounces

QUICK TIP: Add a few drops of your favorite scent to your shower gel, after-bath splash, lotion, and powder. Layering the scent in this way, by using the same scent in all of your products, will create a more intense and longer-lasting fragrance.

Soft to the Touch Overnight Hand Mask

This hand mask is a simple way to soften your hands with hardly any effort. The yogurt is soothing, and all of the oils add plenty of moisture to the skin. Leave it on overnight, and you'll be surprised by how much softer your hands feel the next morning.

2 tablespoons plain yogurt
1 teaspoon castor oil
1/2 teaspoon almond oil
1/2 teaspoon vitamin E oil

Stir all of the ingredients together until you have a creamy lotion.

To use, massage the entire mixture onto your hands, then cover with cotton gloves or socks and leave the mask on overnight. In the morning, wash your hands, then use a rich cream or natural oil to lock in moisture.

Yield: 1 1/2 ounces

Cocoa Cuticle Cream

It's a good idea to use cuticle cream often to condition your cuticles and increase circulation, and this cream will definitely keep your cuticles soft and promote healthy nail growth. Keep a jar of it on your bedside table and massage it into your nails nightly.

2 tablespoons coconut oil
1/2 teaspoon grated cocoa
   butter

Put the coconut oil and cocoa butter in a small microwave-safe container and microwave on low heat just until melted. (You could also do this on the stovetop, preferably in a double boiler. Since it's kind of a pain using a saucepan with such small amounts of ingredients, you might want to make multiple batches at once. To make a smaller batch on the stovetop, place a glass measuring cup inside a pan filled with a few inches of water.) Stir until you have a smooth cream, then pour the cream into a small, clean container. Let it cool completely before using.

To use, massage a small amount into your cuticles.

Yield: 1 ounce

Tough as Nails Oil

If your nails are brittle or prone to breaking or tearing, use this oil to help strengthen them. Castor oil is the most important ingredient in this recipe, since it helps strengthen the nails and cuticles. For an extra boost, put this oil on your nails at night before going to bed; you'll wake up to stronger, more flexible nails. I like to use this oil once or twice a week to keep my nails strong, but you can use it as often as every night.

1 teaspoon light olive oil
1 teaspoon castor oil
¼ teaspoon lemon juice

Pour all of the ingredients into a clean bottle with a tight-fitting lid, and shake to combine. The mixture will tend to separate, so always shake before using.

To use, massage a small amount of the oil into your nails. Leave it on for at least 5 minutes, or even overnight, then wipe off any excess oil.

Yield: ¹/₂ ounce

MANICURE STEP-BY-STEP

Giving yourself a manicure is super simple, and doing it yourself will save you time and money. Here are the basic steps that I follow.

1. **Clean:** Remove all traces of old nail polish if you wear it, then wash your hands.

2. **Soak:** Soften your nails and get them really clean by soaking then for a few minutes in a bowl of warm water with a drop or two of liquid soap stirred in.

3. **Cuticle push:** Apply cuticle cream or a natural oil to the base of your nails and gently push your cuticles back using a cotton swab or wet washcloth.

4. **Trim:** Trim your nails so that they're all the same length and are shaped in squared-off ovals—this is the strongest nail shape.

5. **Hand mask:** Mix up a simple hand mask such as sour cream and honey or natural clay and water, or use one of your favorite facial mask recipes. Spread it all over your hands and leave it on for 10 to 15 minutes, then rinse thoroughly with warm water.

6. **Massage:** Massage a rich cream or natural oil into your hands and nails. If your hands are really dry, cover them with cotton gloves or cotton tube socks and leave the oil and gloves on overnight. You'll wake up with really soft hands. (This is something my grandmother taught me.)

7. **Polish:** Polish your nails, or you can just buff them for a natural shine and to boost circulation and promote healthy nail growth.

Natural Nail Polish

The nail polish found in drugstores is typically packed full of chemical ingredients. This recipe is for those of you who want the look and shine of painted nails, but without the harmful toxins found in regular nail polish. Use the optional henna for a hint of color. It comes in a variety of colors, from red to black.

1 tablespoon light olive oil

1/2 tablespoon white clay powder

1/4 teaspoon red henna powder (optional)

Stir the olive oil and clay together until you have a smooth cream. If the mixture seems too thick, add a bit more olive oil. The mixture should have the consistency of a rich face cream. Stir in the henna if you'd like to add color. Spoon the polish into a small, clean container with a tight-fitting lid.

To use, massage a small amount of the polish into your nails and cuticles. Wipe off any excess with a soft cloth or cotton pad, then buff lightly for a soft natural glow.

Yield: 1/2 ounce

GOOD STUFF: HENNA Henna is made from the leaves of a plant, also called henna, that grows in the Middle East, Africa, and southern Asia. It has been used since at least 4000 BCE to dye the hair, skin, and nails. Ancient mummies have been discovered with fingernails dyed red with henna. Henna is also an excellent hair conditioner and nail strengthener. If you're using it for these purposes, rather than tattoos or as a hair or nail coloring, I recommend neutral or colorless henna—although having red nails like the ancient Egyptians is coming back into style!

Rosy Posey Foot Soak

A foot soak is a great way to relax, and a smart way to start off a pedicure. I love flowers and think it's a nice touch to throw in some petals. Luckily for me, several of my favorites, such as lavender, rose, and marigold, grow around campus. The chamomile contains tannic acid, which can cure and even prevent foot odor. For gift giving, you can package some loose chamomile tea in a nice jar with a tight-fitting lid, along with some dried flowers and a few drops of lavender oil. Tie a floral ribbon around the jar, attach handwritten instructions for use, and include a fresh flower for a special touch.

About 1 gallon hot water
5 chamomile tea bags,
   or 2 tablespoons loose
   chamomile
4 to 6 drops lavender
   essential oil
Flower petals (optional)

Pour the hot water into a small tub, sink, or basin. A size not much larger than your feet is ideal, as the water will be deeper. Add the chamomile and allow it to steep for about 10 minutes. Add the lavender essential oil and the flower petals, then test the temperature to make sure the water isn't too hot. Soak your feet and enjoy!

Yield: 1 treatment

Put Your Best Foot Forward Scrub

My feet get rough and dry very easily, especially during the summer when I tend to spend a lot of time barefoot. This scrub is perfect for smoothing rough heels and getting them really clean.

½ cup rolled oats
½ cup cornmeal
½ cup coarse salt
½ cup light olive oil

Stir all of the ingredients together until you have a thick, grainy mixture. Spoon the scrub into a clean container with a tight-fitting lid and store it in a cool, dry, dark spot, where it will keep for about 4 weeks.

To use, massage about a tablespoon of the mixture into each foot. Leave it on for 5 to 10 minutes, then rinse well with warm water.

Yield: 12 ounces

QUICK TIP: For soft, smooth feet, rub them with a wet pumice stone every time you shower.

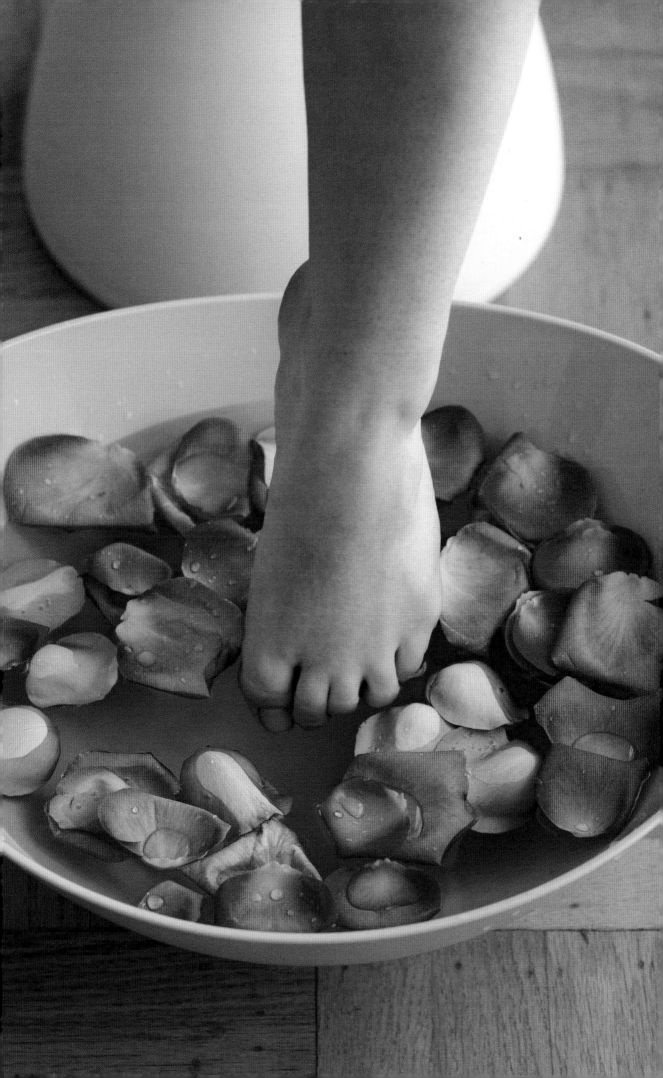

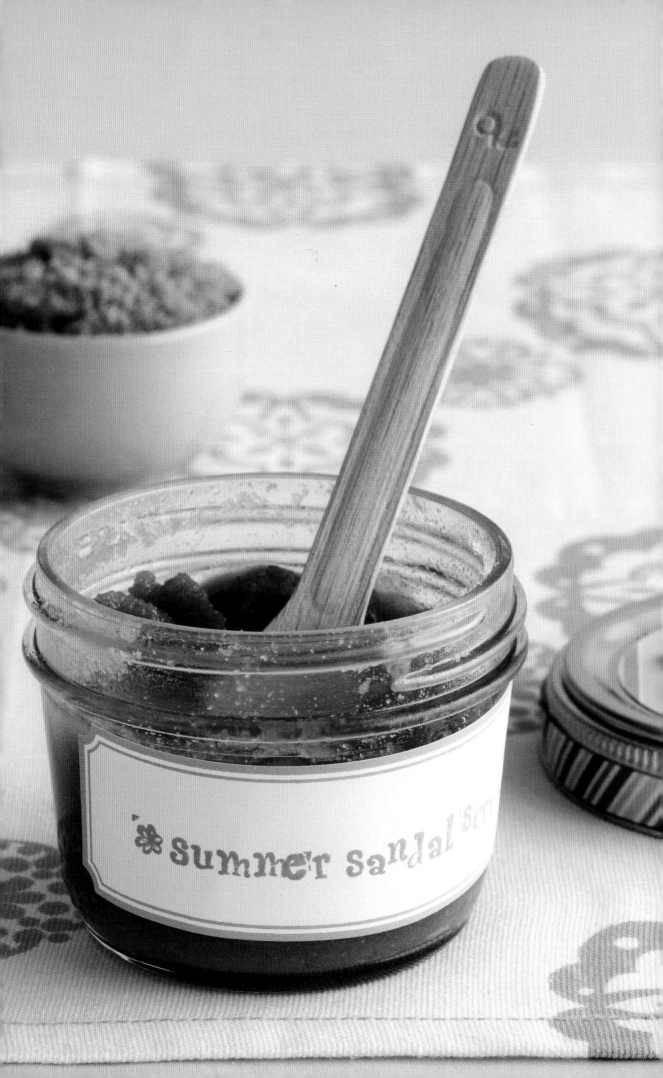

Summer Sandal Scrub

Once sandal season hits, you want your feet to look their best. This scrub will slough off any dead skin. It's a great accompaniment to a home pedicure.

¼ cup brown sugar
2 tablespoons lemon juice
2 tablespoons aloe vera gel
1 teaspoon coconut oil

Stir all of the ingredients together until you have a smooth paste. Store any leftover scrub in a clean jar with a tight-fitting lid in a cool, dry, dark spot. It should last 3 to 4 weeks.

To use, massage 1 to 2 tablespoons of the scrub into each foot, focusing on rough areas, such as your heels.

Yield: 3 ounces

CITRUS PEDI

Soak your feet in a basin of warm water with a couple cups of orange juice added. After soaking for 5 minutes, scrub your feet with ½ cup sugar, then rinse well with warm water and pat your feet dry. Your toes will thank you!

PEDICURE STEP-BY-STEP

Few things are worse than wanting to wear a pair of strappy sandals or flip-flops and having your feet look a mess. Here are the steps I follow to quickly shape up my feet.

1. **Clean and soften:** Remove all old nail polish if you wear it, then soak your feet in a small tub or basin filled with warm water with a cup of white vinegar or pineapple juice added. The acidic water will help clean and soften your feet.

2. **Scrub:** Use a pumice stone or salt scrub to really clean your feet and smooth any rough or tough skin.

3. **Trim:** Trim your toenails. (Doing this after soaking makes for a cleaner cut.) Cut the nails straight across to avoid ingrown toenails.

4. **Mask:** Mix up a rich mask of green clay and peppermint oil (2 tablespoons of clay with 1 to 2 tablespoons of water and 4 to 5 drops of peppermint oil should do the trick). Spread the mask onto your feet to soften and clean them. Leave it on for 10 to 15 minutes, then rinse thoroughly with warm water and pat your feet dry.

5. **Massage:** Massage a rich cream or body butter into your feet and toenails, then gently push back the cuticle at the base of each nail.

High Heel Foot Spray

Sometimes you just have to wear high heels; not only are they perfect for certain outfits, they're also simply fun to wear. But after I spend a day or an evening in them, my feet definitely need some TLC. This spray helps energize tired feet and also fights any foot odor. Just spray some on and you'll have happy feet that want to jump for joy! I have a friend who's a prima ballerina, so you can imagine the workout her feet get. She loves this recipe.

1 cup distilled water

½ teaspoon tea tree oil

5 drops peppermint essential oil

Pour all of the ingredients into a spray bottle and shake to combine.

To use, spray the mixture onto your feet for a quick pick-me-up.

Yield: 8 ounces

Extreme Makeover Foot Edition

Want instantly softer feet? This overnight treatment is the easiest way to get them. The cocoa butter will hydrate your feet, and the aloe vera will help repair any damage to the skin. When you wake up in the morning, your feet will be dramatically softer.

½ cup rolled oats

3 tablespoons grated cocoa butter

3 tablespoons honey

2 tablespoons aloe vera gel

Stir all of the ingredients together until you have a smooth paste.

To use, massage all of the mixture onto your feet, then wrap your feet in plastic wrap and put on cotton socks. Leave the treatment on overnight. Be careful not to make a mess when removing everything the next morning, then rinse your feet thoroughly with warm water and pat your feet dry.

Yield: 4–5 ounces

QUICK TIP: For smooth feet, massage a rich natural oil such as coconut oil or dark sesame oil into them at night, then put on a pair of cotton socks and leave the oil on overnight. You'll wake up with super soft feet.

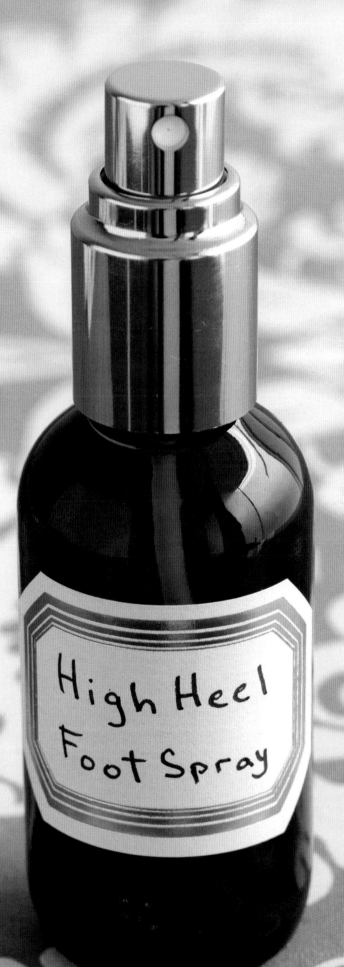

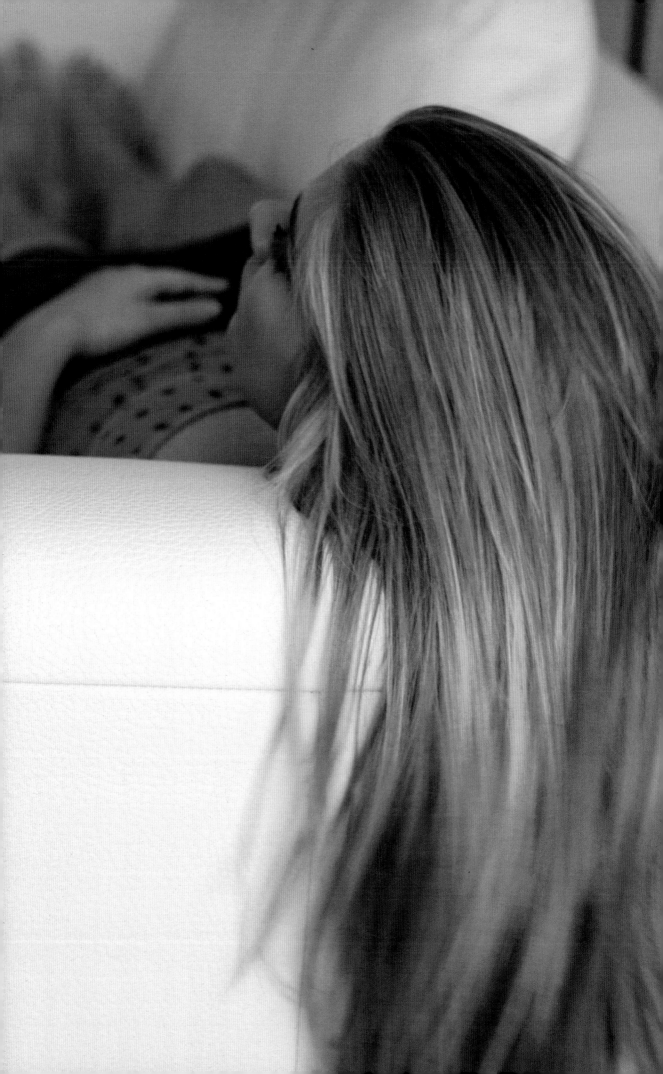

FOR THE HAIR

Hair is an important part of a person's identity and look. Whether yours is curly, straight, short, or long, how you wear your hair says a lot about who you are. Today hairstyles are more fun and casual than ever before, and when it comes to cut, color, and length, just about anything goes. The state of your hair can also say a lot about how you feel. We've all heard the expression "bad hair day." I hate it when my hair just won't cooperate and I just have to tie it up in a ponytail. My sister is a bit more daring with her hairstyles, and she is always experimenting with twisted updos and braids.

Hair, like skin, does require special care. It's important to keep it clean, well conditioned, and protected from the elements.

Cleansing products like shampoo are intended primarily to clean your scalp. A clean, healthy scalp will lead to healthy hair. So really focus on your scalp when washing your hair. Some people wash their hair every day, and others every other day. This is really a matter of personal choice, as you know best what works for you. Traditional shampoos are full of soap and make a lot of lather, but there's a new trend to use natural oils to condition and cleanse the scalp and hair, and these tend to foam less. Again, what you choose to use is a matter of personal choice and hair type; just make sure that it keeps your scalp clean so you can avoid greasy roots and dandruff.

Conditioners and hair masks are great for restoring lost moisture, which is especially important if you dye your hair or use a lot of heated styling tools, such as curlers, straighteners, and blow-dryers. I like to treat my hair to a deep conditioning honey hair mask once a week; it really works to rehydrate my hair and keep it healthy and flexible. If you pluck a hair from your scalp and pull on it gently, it should stretch and be pretty hard to break. If it breaks easily, it's too dry and needs conditioning!

Hair rinses are another easy treatment to add to your hair care regime. They can be used to highlight, cleanse, or condition your hair. Many hairdressers recommend using a baking soda rinse monthly to get your hair super clean and avoid any buildup of styling products. This is good advice; it's amazing how well baking soda eats through old hair spray, styling gels, and leave-in conditioners.

Styling products are also easy to make, and of course they're fun to use. You can create your own scented hair oils and gels and even hair sprays that are just as effective as commercial products.

ECO TIP: Choose hair salons that are eco-friendly for cuts and trims. An eco-friendly salon is an environmentally friendly, nontoxic place to get beautiful. They recycle, use chemical-free hair dyes and treatments, use pumps rather than aerosol products, and clean with biodegradable products. They also often have very costly ventilation systems to rid the salon of harmful dust and fumes. If you're not sure, just ask!

TEN TIPS FOR AWESOME HAIR

Having healthy, shiny tresses is something that will get you noticed. Here are ten simple steps to keep your locks manageable and full of shine:

1. Keep your hair trimmed. You should schedule a trim or haircut every six to eight weeks.

2. Treat yourself to a weekly deep conditioning treatment or hair mask.

3. Wear a swimming cap and rinse your hair well after swimming in the ocean or a pool.

4. Massage your scalp to boost circulation and promote hair growth.

5. Use a cleansing baking soda rinse monthly to rid your hair of any buildup.

6. Keep your brushes, combs, curlers, and heated styling equipment clean.

7. Avoid the high heat setting on blow-dryers, flat irons, and curling irons.

8. Wear a hat to protect your hair from sun and wind when you're outdoors.

9. For soft natural curls and waves, sleep in braids or old-fashioned pin curls at night.

10. Change your ponytail position often to avoid breakage.

Basic Shampoo

This is a great basic shampoo for all hair types. If your hair is oily, omit the optional vegetable oil, but if your hair is dry or damaged, you should definitely include it. This shampoo is gentle on hair and won't strip away its natural oils, so it will help keep your hair healthy and shiny.

½ cup water
½ cup liquid soap
½ teaspoon light vegetable oil (leave out for oily hair)

Gently stir all of the ingredients together, being careful not to beat the mixture, as this will cause it to foam up. Pour the shampoo into a clean squeeze bottle or plastic container.

To use, shampoo as you normally would, then rinse well with cool water.

Yield: 8 ounces

ECO TIP: Turn the water off while you're lathering up shampoo in your hair. You can save more than fifty gallons of water per week this way.

Honey Hair Pack

Honey and molasses are both humectants, meaning they attract and hold onto water molecules. This makes them great ingredients for adding moisture to the hair. If your hair is a bit on the oily side, you can leave out the olive oil. But no matter what your hair type, this elixir will help condition your hair cuticles, resulting in shiny, smooth hair.

½ cup honey or molasses
1 tablespoon extra-virgin olive oil

Stir the honey and oil together until well mixed.

To use, apply the entire mixture to your head (with your hair dry) and massage it into your hair and scalp. Put on a shower cap or cover your hair with plastic wrap and leave the treatment on for 20 to 30 minutes, then wash and condition your hair as usual.

Yield: 4½ ounces

ECO TIP: Install a low-flow showerhead in your shower stall to save water and money.

Lightening Hair Rinse

This rinse works best for blond or light brown hair. With repeated use, it will subtly lighten the color of your hair and bring out natural highlights. Fresh rhubarb may be hard to find year-round, but you can also use frozen.

4 cups water

1/2 cup chopped rhubarb

5 chamomile tea bags,
   or 2 tablespoons dried
   chamomile leaves and
   flowers

1 teaspoon borax

Bring the water, rhubarb, and tea to a boil, then remove from the heat and let steep for at least 20 to 30 minutes. Once the mixture is completely cool, strain or remove the rhubarb and tea bag, then add the borax. Store any remaining rinse in the refrigerator, where it should keep for 3 to 4 weeks.

To use, massage one cup of the hair rinse into your clean, damp hair after shampooing, and don't rinse it out. For an extra boost, after applying the rinse go out in the sun and let your hair dry naturally.

Yield: 4 treatments

Refreshing Mint Hair Rinse

If you're in need of a refreshing pick-me-up for dull, limp locks, this rinse will do the trick. Together, the mint tea and vinegar will get your scalp really clean and leave your hair fresh and shiny. Mint is naturally energizing and will give your scalp a tingly, fresh feeling, and the vinegar will rid your hair of any residue from styling gels or soap-based shampoos.

1/2 cup boiling water

1 to 2 mint tea bags

2 tablespoons apple cider
   vinegar

Pour the boiling water over the tea bag and let it steep until cool. Remove the tea bag, pressing it to extract as much tea as possible, then stir in the vinegar.

To use, shampoo and condition your hair as usual, then apply the entire mixture to your hair. Massage it into your scalp and work it through your hair, then dry your hair as you normally would, without rinsing it out.

Yield: 4 ounces

Under the Sea Hair Rinse

There is a reason why mermaids always seem to have a gorgeous mane of hair: seaweed! This rinse will strengthen your hair and make it instantly shinier and smoother. Plus, many people believe that kelp helps promote hair growth.

$^1/_2$ **cup water**

$^1/_2$ **cup apple cider vinegar**

$^1/_4$ **cup lemon juice**

2 tablespoons powdered kelp

Stir all of the ingredients together until well mixed. Pour the rinse into a clean bottle or container.

To use, first shampoo your hair, then coat your damp hair with the entire mixture. Put on a shower cap or wrap your hair in an old towel and leave the treatment on for 20 minutes, then rinse your hair thoroughly.

Yield: 10 ounces

QUICK AND EASY HAIR RINSES

Here are a few of my favorite hair rinses. Simply pour the mixture on your hair after shampooing and comb it through.

❋ **Cleansing:** Put a teaspoon of baking soda into a cup of water and stir until dissolved.

❋ **Shine enhancing:** Stir a teaspoon of apple cider vinegar into a cup of water.

❋ **Highlighting:** Brew some strong chamomile tea, using several tea bags in a cup of hot water; let it cool to a comfortable temperature before applying. Another option is a teaspoon of lemon juice mixed into a cup of water.

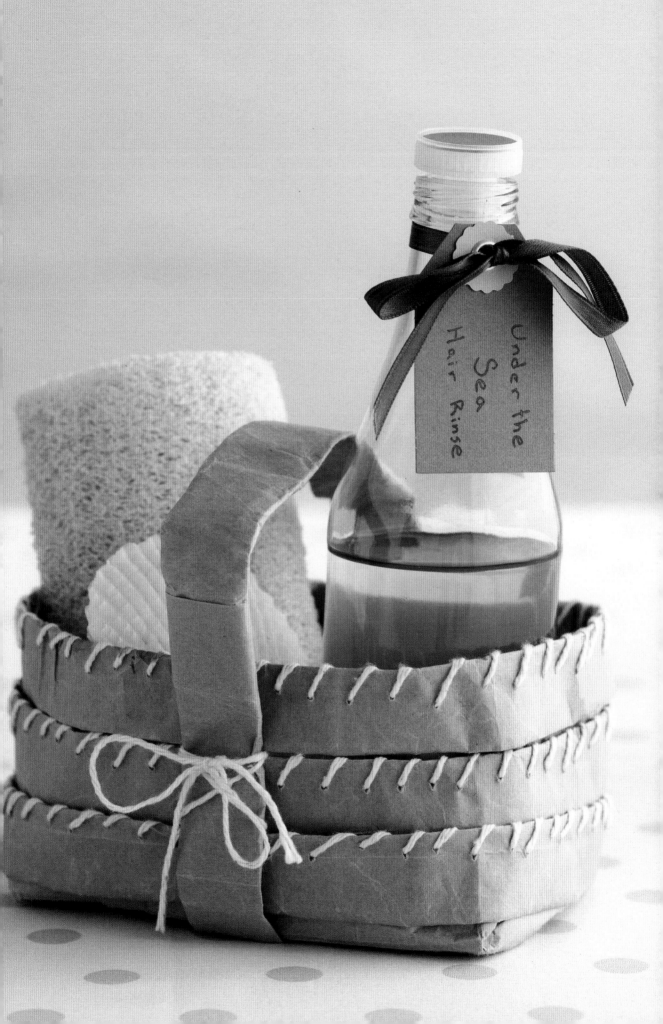

Clay Hair Mask

If you have oily hair, a clay hair mask is a great option. French green clay is the best for the job, because it's so effective at extracting toxins and oils from the scalp. If your scalp is already dry, this isn't the treatment for you.

¼ cup natural clay powder
2 tablespoons mineral water
½ teaspoon cider vinegar

Stir all of the ingredients together until you have a smooth paste.

To use, apply the entire mixture to clean, damp hair and massage it into your scalp and hair. Put on a shower cap or cover your hair with plastic wrap and leave the mask on for 10 to 15 minutes, then rinse well with warm water. You may need to rinse your hair for several minutes to remove all of the clay.

Yield: 2 ounces

ECO TIP: When shopping for ingredients such as herbs, clay, and spices, buy in bulk to save both packaging and money.

911 Hair Rescue Mask

This great hair conditioning mask for repairing dry, damaged hair is especially good if you use a lot of high-heat styling tools, such as a blow-dryer or straightening iron. It will help revive lackluster hair, from your scalp to the ends of your hair.

½ cup plain yogurt
2 tablespoons light olive oil
3 to 4 drops essential oil of peppermint
1 to 2 drops essential oil of rosemary or 1 sprig fresh rosemary

Put all of the ingredients in a blender or food processor and blend until you have a smooth mixture.

To use, first shampoo your hair, then apply the entire mixture and massage it into your hair and scalp. Put on a shower cap or wrap your hair in an old towel and leave the mixture on for 15 to 20 minutes, then rinse well with warm water and style as usual.

Yield: 5 ounces

Pre-Shampoo Hair Conditioner

The purpose of conditioner is to keep hair nourished and tamed, and this great basic conditioner will leave your locks shiny and smooth. Because this conditioner is so rich and full of natural oils, it is best to use it before shampooing so that you do not end up with oily hair. For a deeper conditioning effect, apply it to dry hair and let it sit for about 5 minutes. Save the leftover egg white to use in Milk Maid Cleanser (page 17), Fresh Strawberry Mask (page 24), or Hollywood Bubble Bath (page 66); if you won't be using it right away, just store it in the freezer.

1 tablespoon lemon juice
1 tablespoon honey
1 teaspoon almond oil
1 teaspoon avocado oil
1 teaspoon olive oil
1 egg yolk

Stir all of the ingredients together until well mixed.

To use, apply the entire mixture to your head (with your hair dry) and massage it into your hair and scalp. Put on a shower cap or wrap your hair in plastic wrap and leave the conditioner on for 15 minutes, then shampoo your hair as usual and rinse well.

Yield: 2 ounces

Dandruff Treatment

One night I was dressed up and ready to go out in one of my favorite little black dresses. Then to my horror I noticed dandruff on the shoulders of my dress! I changed into something else, and as soon as I got home that night I mixed up this treatment to get rid of my dandruff as quickly as possible. Dandruff is a sign of a dry scalp that needs to be rehydrated or conditioned. The apple cider or lemon juice helps cleanse your scalp and rid it of any loose, dry flakes of skin. The olive oil moisturizes the skin on your head and helps lock in moisture.

2 tablespoons apple cider
   vinegar or lemon juice
2 tablespoons distilled water
2 tablespoons light or
   extra-virgin olive oil

Stir all of the ingredients together until well mixed.

To use, apply the entire mixture to damp hair and thoroughly massage it into your scalp. Leave the treatment on for 20 minutes, then shampoo and condition as usual.

Yield: 3 ounces

Avocado Hair Conditioner

When your hair is super dry or damaged, you need a deep conditioner. Avocados, which are rich in oil, protein, B vitamins, and vitamin A, will definitely do the trick. They contain more protein than any other fruit, and their abundant natural oil will coat your hair and form a protective barrier, keeping your hair well hydrated, soft, and flexible. For ultimate self-indulgence, sip a hot cup of tea while your hair soaks up this nourishing mask.

1 ripe avocado, mashed
2 tablespoons sour cream
  or plain yogurt
Juice of ½ lemon

Stir all of the ingredients together until you have a smooth paste; either a fork or a blender will work well.

To use, apply the entire mixture to your head (with your hair dry) and massage it into your hair and scalp. Wrap your hair in a warm towel or put on a shower cap and leave the treatment on for 20 minutes. Rinse well with warm water, then shampoo as usual.

Yield: 2 ounces

QUICK TIP: Save the avocado pit! You can use it as a massage tool or grind it up to use in a body scrub.

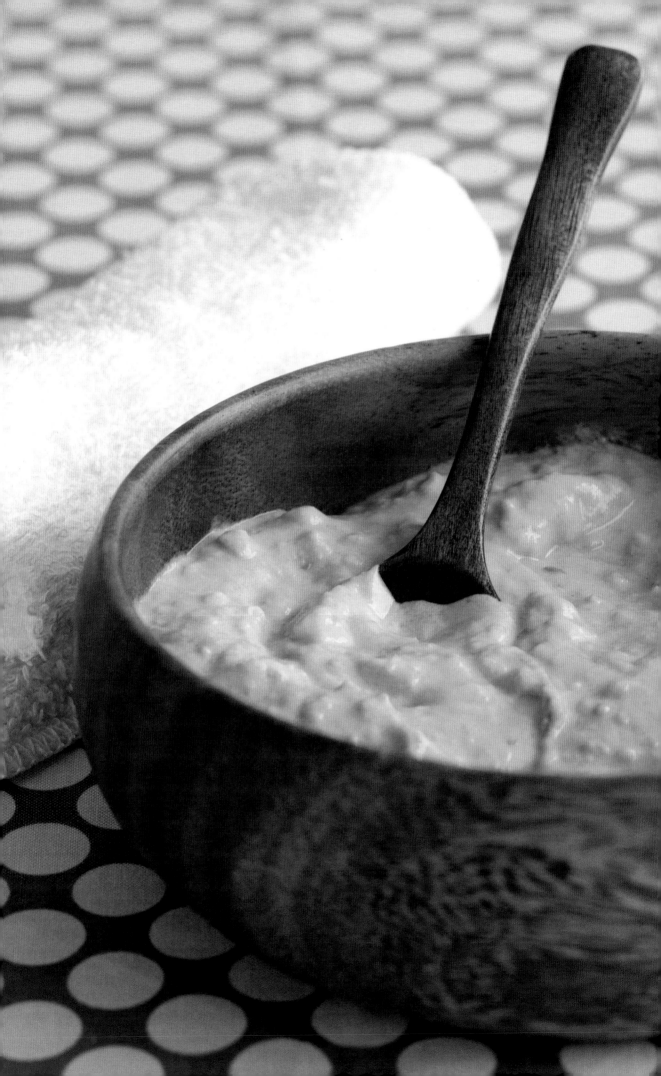

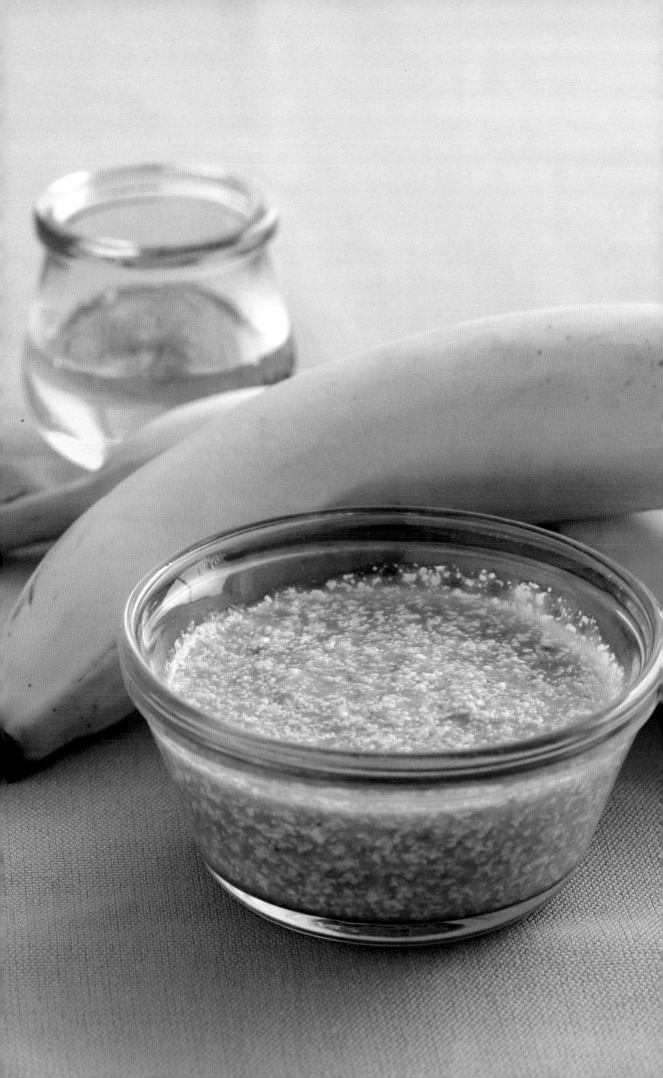

Go Bananas Hair Conditioner

Bananas are great for conditioning hair deeply and moisturizing the scalp. This recipe will make your hair very manageable and leave it smelling like you've just returned from a tropical island paradise. Very ripe bananas work best in this recipe. Make sure you blend the mixture until it's really smooth; this will make it easier to rinse out.

$^1/_2$ ripe banana

$^1/_4$ cup warm water

2 tablespoons honey

1 teaspoon coconut oil

Mash the banana, then put it in a blender, add the water, honey, and coconut oil, and blend until very smooth. (You can also do this by hand, but a blender works better.)

To use, first shampoo your hair, then apply the entire mixture to your hair and massage it into your hair and scalp. Wrap a warm towel around your head or put on a shower cap and leave the treatment on for about 30 minutes, then rinse your hair thoroughly.

Yield: 4 ounces

Hot Oil Treatment

This is the ultimate treatment for dry and damaged hair. It will put plenty of moisture back into stressed tresses. Honey has a mild bleaching effect over time, so if you have color-treated or darker hair I suggest using dark molasses in this recipe. Do this right before bathing or showering because the warmer the oil stays, the more effective the treatment. Just be careful that you don't slip in the shower while rinsing it out!

$^1/_4$ cup almond oil

1 tablespoon honey or dark
    molasses, depending on
    hair type

Put the oil and honey in a microwave-safe container and microwave on high heat until warm to touch, about 30 seconds. Alternatively, you can warm the mixture in a small saucepan on the stovetop. Stir the warm mixture until thoroughly combined.

To use, apply the entire mixture to dry hair and massage it into your hair and scalp. Wrap your hair in a warm towel or put on a shower cap and leave the treatment on for up to 30 minutes, then rinse thoroughly with warm water and shampoo as usual.

Yield: 2$^1/_2$ ounces

Beach Babe Hair Spray

Salty sea breeze spritzes and sprays seem to be all the rage. They give your hair that casual "I just spent all day at the beach" look. Salt sprays are also used to give your hair texture and natural waves. However, they can be drying, so try to limit how often you use them, and use a good hair conditioning pack weekly to keep your hair soft and flexible.

1 cup warm water

2 to 3 tablespoons sea salt

1 to 2 drops essential oil (optional)

Put all of the ingredients in a clean spray bottle and shake vigorously until the salt dissolves.

To use, while drying and tousling your hair, spray it with this recipe to build volume and create that "fresh from a day at the beach" look.

Yield: 8 ounces

CALIFORNIA BEACH HAIR

I go to school in Southern California, where everyone loves going to the beach. Here are some simple tips to keep your hair looking its best while hitting the sand:

* Cover up with a scarf or hat to protect your hair from the sun and wind.

* Comb a rich conditioner through your hair while you're at the beach and leave it on. The heat from the sun will boost its conditioning power.

* For natural highlights, spray your hair with chamomile tea or lemon water while you're at the beach.

* Rinse your hair with fresh water after swimming, since salt water can be drying. In fact, you may want to bring an extra water bottle for this purpose.

* Braid your hair while it's wet, and you'll have natural waves once it's dry.

* Remember, you can get a sunburn on your scalp, so use sunscreen on the part in your hair.

ECO TIP: I make hair ties and hair bands out of old nylons and tights. For hair ties, simply cut rings out of the legs and use them to hold your hair in place. For hair bands, I cut long strips and braid them into a band. After making sure it fits around my head, I stitch the ends together. These work really well at keeping your hair in place, and they won't damage or break your hair. Plus, it's a great way to reuse a pair of tights that have a run.

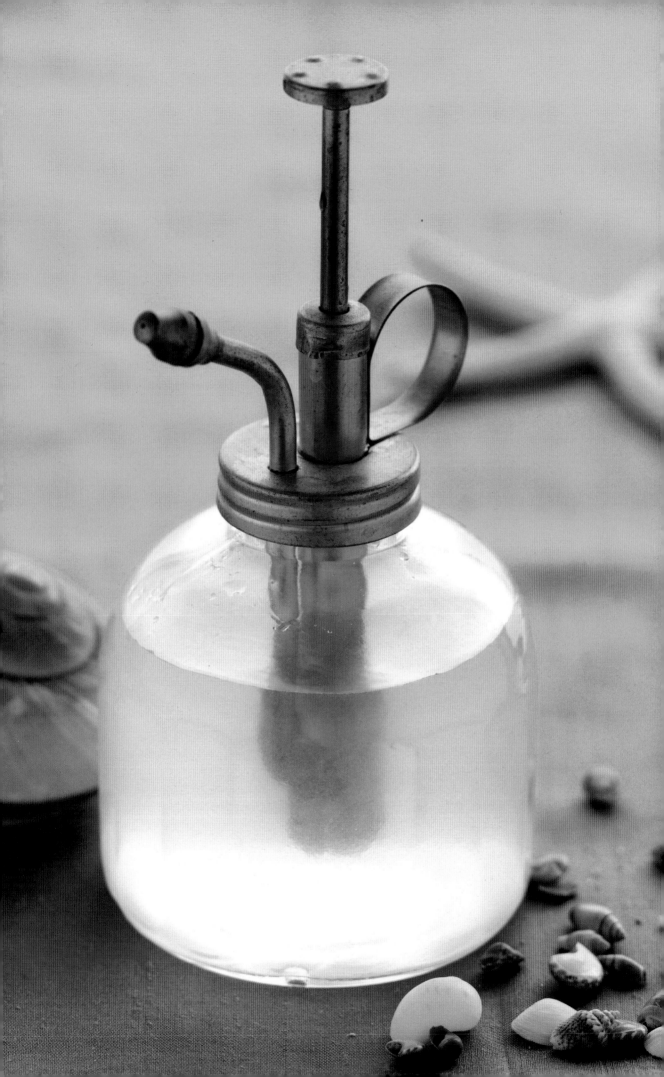

Swimming Pool Hair Care

One of my best friends worked as a lifeguard over the summer. She soon learned that the chlorine gave her gorgeous blond hair a green tint. She asked me what she should do, and I passed along this recipe. In no time at all, her beautiful natural hair color was completely restored.

¼ cup lemon juice

2 tablespoons baking soda

1 teaspoon mild shampoo or liquid soap, such as baby shampoo or castile soap

Stir all of the ingredients together until well mixed.

To use, wet your hair, apply the entire mixture, then massage it into your hair and scalp, making sure the ends of your hair are coated. Put on a shower cap or cover your hair with plastic wrap and leave the treatment on for 30 minutes, then rinse your hair well and shampoo and condition as usual.

Yield: 2 ounces

BEAUTY SMARTS: WHY DOES POOL WATER TURN YOUR HAIR GREEN? Pool water often has a high concentration of copper, which tends to turn light-colored hair green over time. The copper can come from a number of sources, from the water supply to the pipes. The copper deposit actually forms on other colors of hair too—it's just most noticeable on blond hair.

Voluptuous Volume Spray

For a night out, sometimes I prefer big teased hair to my usual sleek look. This spray helps create volume in my hair and thicken it at the roots. All I need to top it off is some teasing and a little hairspray.

3/4 cup water

3 tablespoons white vinegar

2 tablespoons honey

Pour all of the ingredients into a spray bottle and shake to thoroughly combine.

To use, spray it onto damp hair and work it through from the root to ends. Don't rinse it out; just style your hair as usual.

Yield: 8 1/2 ounces

Styling Gel

Making your own styling gel is a great way to save some money. This version works just as well as what you might buy, but it costs only pennies to make. You can scent your gel using a few drops of a favorite essential oil. This recipe also makes a great gift for your favorite guy friend who could use a little styling help. Pick a "macho" scent such as bay, sage, or allspice.

1 cup water

1 teaspoon unflavored gelatin

1 to 2 drops essential oil
   (optional)

Heat the water but don't bring it to a boil. Stir in the gelatin and the essential oil. Pour the mixture into a clean container with a tight-fitting lid, and let it set up before using it. Stored in the refrigerator, the gel will keep for about 4 weeks. If you use it every day, you can store it in a cool, dry, dark place like a bathroom cabinet.

To use, apply the gel as you would any styling gel, to add body to your hair and help hold it in place.

Yield: 8 ounces

ECO TIP: Did you know that a blow-dryer uses more energy than a vacuum? Air-dry your hair at least once a week to save energy—and to save your hair!

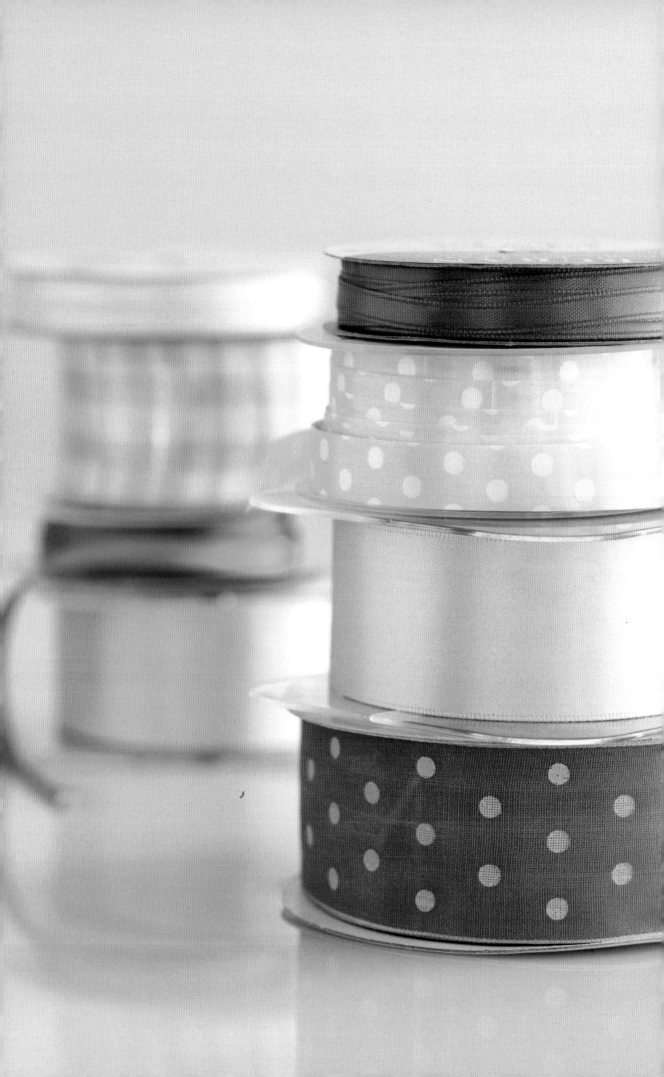

GIFT GIVING

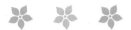

I've always loved making gifts for my friends and family. For me, it's relaxing, fun, and saves a bunch of money. It's also a great way to create unique and personal presents. Homemade beauty products make great gifts. Not only are they really easy to make, they're useful and everyone loves them. Most people can always use a new lip balm, scrub, or rich body butter.

I love to put together festive baskets for holidays and special occasions. You can also make theme baskets to give to your friends before a big test or a special date, or before they head off to college. They'll appreciate it! I know I can always use some antistress therapy and pampering during my first week back at school.

Creating fun packaging and labels is almost as much fun as making the products themselves. I've made gift containers out of buckets, paper sacks, newspaper, cereal boxes, and old vinyl records. You can also have fun naming all of your products, and these days digital cameras and computer software make it a snap to customize just about everything from stickers to CD labels. I've even put laminated digital photos inside bars of homemade glycerin soap. Most of all, I like the good karma you get from giving. I truly do believe that it's better to give than to receive, and being thoughtful is always a good idea. So have fun and be creative!

FUN BASKET IDEAS

Putting together gift baskets for friends and family is so rewarding. Coming up with the theme can be as much fun as filling them, and there's no limit to what you can do. Start with a fun container. Use your imagination; it can be a basket, a small bucket, a Chinese take-out container, or something repurposed from another use. Fill the bottom of the container with some shredded paper or colored tissue paper. Doing this keeps it from weighing a ton; plus, you won't need as much stuff to make it look really full. Then arrange the gifts in the basket, and don't forget to tie it up with a big bow. Here are some theme baskets I've put together:

Happy foot basket: When my friends who play sports or dance have a big game or show, I like to give them this basket. Fill a plastic tub large enough for a foot bath with pedicure tools, a new pumice stone, Energizing Leg Gel (page 53), and fresh lemons to cut in half and use for softening rough skin spots. Include a handwritten note of encouragement or congratulations.

Workout basket: If someone you know is starting a new exercise routine or needs a bit of motivation, make them a CD with workout tunes and put it in a small gym bag, along with water bottles, shower gel, body powder, and Energizing Bath Bombs (page 131).

Birthday basket: Put together a basket of body care items and encourage your friend to take time to pamper herself on her special day. I always include Cupcake Bath Bombs (page 132), lip balms, enough white clay for a year's worth of facial masks, a new bright washcloth, and Mardi Gras beads or handmade beads made from magazine paper (see sidebar, page 139).

Keep smiling: When my sister got braces, I put together a small bag full of soothing mouth care products: Minty Toothpaste (page 87), Apple Juice Mouth Rinse (page 88), Chocolate Brownie Lip Gloss (page 85), and a bright, new, soft toothbrush. It made her smile!

Bon voyage: When my friends travel and need to adjust to a new time zone, I always give them two little bottles of essential oil: peppermint for energy and lavender to help them go to sleep. Because the bottles are so small, they're easy to pack and even get through airport security—which is no small feat these days.

HOLIDAY GIFTS

Holidays are the perfect time for homemade gifts. Here are some of my favorite ideas to help you share some holiday joy!

❋ **Halloween:** Not everyone wants to look their best on Halloween. Luckily, green clay can be used either way. I love to package it up with a funny saying like "Have a boo-tiful day!" and give it to all of my friends. This way they can look scary for a while but have really great skin afterward.

❋ **Thanksgiving:** If you're a houseguest, homemade pumpkin spice bath salts make a great hostess gift. Just add a teaspoon of pumpkin pie spice to 1 cup of Epsom salts and ½ cup of baking soda. They're also a nice way to thank your mom for making your favorite sweet potato casserole.

❋ **Christmas:** This is a fun time to make stocking stuffers such as bath bombs, lip balms, gift soaps, and bath salts (peppermint scented, of course). You can make your own holiday stockings to hold them all, or just use a cute gift bag decorated with a holiday theme.

❋ **Hanukkah:** Small presents are perfect for Hanukkah. In addition to the traditional chocolate coins and dreidels, you can also give a pretty jar of homemade rich body butter. You can also make some quick and easy scented bath oil by adding a few drops of your favorite essential oil to a cup of light sesame or almond oil and pouring it into a cute bottle.

❋ **Valentine's Day:** I only have one word for you: *chocolate*. Fill a heart-shaped box or a box decorated with hearts with Chocolate Brownie Lip Gloss (page 85), Chocolate Massage Butter (page 50), and, of course, some chocolates kisses!

❋ **Easter:** Easter signals the end of winter and the beginning of spring—a time when most people could use some extra pampering since winter can be hard on the skin and we all want to look good in spring outfits. Use plastic eggs to mold bath bombs, adding a few drops of food coloring or all-natural alternative (see sidebar, page 65) to the bath bomb mixture to make them pretty pastel colors.

❋ **Fourth of July:** Create a fun red, white, and blue beach basket that will pamper your friend after a day at the beach or a weekend of camping. Include a jar of Mermaid Skin Scrub (page 23), some Colored Bath Salts (page 128), Summer Sandal Scrub (page 103), a jar of coconut oil for moisturizing dry skin, and aloe vera gel just in case of sunburn. You can also include bandanas, beach hats, and a new aluminum water bottle to make sure your friend stays well hydrated.

Colored Bath Salts

You can create dozens of different bath salts in no time at all. All you need is a combination of natural salts, such as Epsom salts, sea salt, and kosher salt, and some food coloring—look for the pastel varieties used in cake decorating, or investigate natural sources of color (see sidebar, page 65). You can also scent your salts. The result will be a gift to rival any store-bought bath salt. There used to be a kiosk at our local mall where you could choose your salt, color, and scent, and they would mix it up on the spot and package it in a Chinese take-out box. The funny thing was, they were using one of my mom's recipes—and charging dollars for what we made at home for pennies. But then again, rent is pretty high at the mall.

1 cup Epsom salts
½ cup rock salt or kosher salt
3 to 5 drops food coloring
4 to 5 drops essential oil

Stir all of the ingredients together until well mixed. I like to do this in a large plastic resealable bag, as you can seal it and massage the mixture until the color and scent are evenly distributed. Check out the color and add more food coloring if you like, or, if the color is too dark add more salt. Pour the bath salts into a clean jar or pretty gift container.

To use, pour about ½ cup of bath salts under running water while drawing a bath. Relax in the tub and enjoy!

Yield: 12 ounces

BATH SALT IDEAS

Once you start making bath salts, you'll have so much fun thinking up new scents, colors, and gift combinations. Here are some of my best ideas:

Herbal: For a natural-looking herbal bath salt, skip the color and add a tablespoon or two of your favorite dried herbs. I like to use lavender, thyme, mint, or rosemary. You can also use a combination of herbs, or flower petals like calendula and rose.

Candy: For holiday bath salts, add a few small seasonal candies to the jar (but not chocolates!). For example, you can add candy conversation hearts for Valentine's Day or candy corn for Halloween. They look cute in the jar and will easily melt in the tub. Plus, sugar is a good skin softener.

Layers: Mix up several batches of different colors of bath salt and layer them in glass containers for a cool striped effect. For Christmas, I like to make batches of red and white bath salts with a few drops of peppermint essential oil or peppermint extract, then layer them in the jar so it looks like a big candy cane.

Moisturizing: When combining the ingredients, add a tablespoon of your favorite light oil for a moisturizing blend.

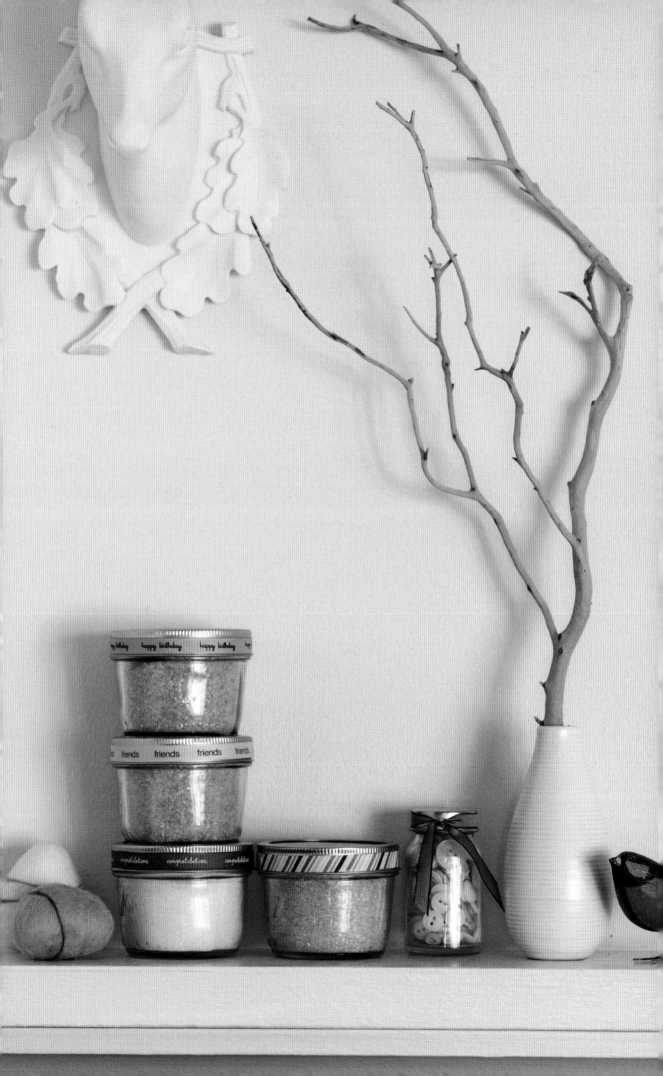

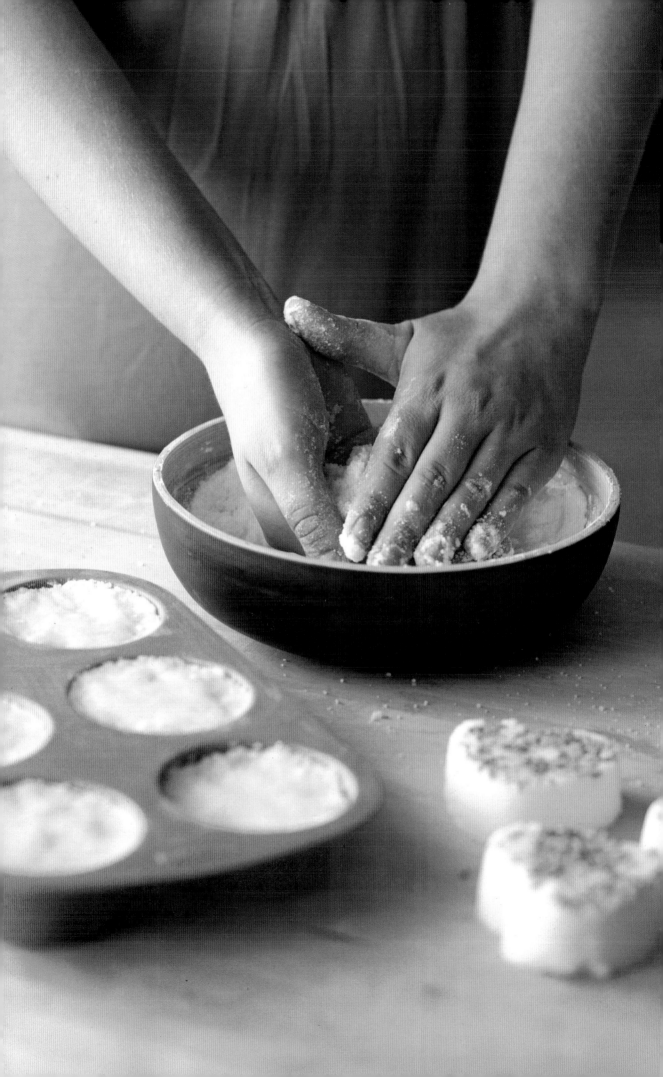

Moisturizing Bath Bombs

This is a great gift to give during the winter months, when dry skin is on the rise. I like to use heart-shape molds and give them during chilly February as Valentine's Day gifts—you can put candy hearts on top, or sprinkle them with lavender for a more natural look. These bath bombs will not only add moisture to the tub but also help skin retain moisture and feel silky soft. Check out Shower Gel Scents (see page 70) for some suggestions on scents to create different moods.

1 cup baking soda

1 cup citric acid powder

$1/2$ cup cornstarch

$1/2$ cup light oil, such as almond, canola, or sunflower

1 teaspoon vitamin E oil

10 to 12 drops essential oil (optional)

Plastic molds such as ice cube trays, candy molds, or muffin tins

Stir all of the ingredients together until you have a crumbly dough. The mixture will seem pretty crumbly, but it should hold together. Pack the mixture into the molds and let the bath bombs set up overnight. The next day, gently tap the mold to release the bath bombs, then let them air-dry for a day.

To use, drop one bath bomb into a warm tub and enjoy!

Yield: 16 ounces, approximately 4 bath bombs

Energizing Bath Bombs

When you add these bath bombs to the tub, the combination of citric acid and baking soda makes them fizz and "explode." They're so fun to use, and fun to give as gifts, too. I love how you can change their bathing effect just by using a few different ingredients. This recipe is especially energizing because of the peppermint extract. It has a fresh, clean scent that will really boost your mood and your energy level. And needless to say, it's much better for your body than energy drinks.

1 cup baking soda

1 cup citric acid powder

$1/2$ cup cornstarch

$1/2$ cup light oil, such as almond, canola, or sunflower

1 teaspoon peppermint extract

2 to 3 drops green food coloring (optional)

Plastic molds, such as ice cube trays, candy molds, or muffin tins

Stir all of the ingredients together until you have a crumbly dough. The mixture will seem pretty crumbly, but it should hold together. If it seems too oily add more baking soda, and if it seems too dry add a small amount of oil. Pack the mixture into the molds and let the bath bombs set up overnight. The next day, gently tap the molds to release the bath bombs, then let them air-dry for a day.

To use, drop one bath bomb into a warm tub and enjoy!

Yield: 16 ounces, approximately 4 bath bombs

Cupcake Bath Bombs

These bath bombs make the most adorable gifts for birthdays and holidays. You can even make up a bunch to give out as party favors. I have fun tinting the "frosting" with different colors (see the sidebar on page 65 for natural color options), then decorating them with candy sprinkles. Don't worry; the sprinkles will dissolve in the tub. Another option is to decorate the top of each bath bomb with a hard candy, which will also melt in the tub. If you do it up, these bath bombs will look just like real cupcakes, but instead of being loaded with calories, they contain plenty of oil to help nourish your skin.

1 cup baking soda

1 cup citric acid powder

$^1/_2$ cup cornstarch

$^1/_2$ cup light oil, such as almond, canola, or sunflower

Plastic or silicon cupcake molds or paper liners

2 to 3 drops food coloring

Small candies or sprinkles

Mix the baking soda, citric acid powder, cornstarch, and oil until you have a crumbly dough. Reserve $^1/_2$ cup of the mixture for the "frosting" and pack the rest of the mixture into cupcake molds. Color the reserved mixture with the food coloring, and pat an equal amount atop each cupcake. Decorate each cupcake with a few candy sprinkles. Let the cupcakes set up overnight. The next day, gently tap the mold to release the cupcakes, being careful not to disturb the decorations, then let them air-dry for a day.

To use, drop one bath bomb into a warm tub and enjoy!

Yield: 16 ounces, approximately 4 bath bombs

$HOPPING TIP: CITRIC ACID POWDER Citric acid powder can be found in the section of the grocery store that carries ingredients and supplies for canning foods. I sometimes use all-natural pectin; just be sure to check the label and verify that citric acid is listed as the main ingredient. You can also purchase bags of citric acid powder at natural food stores and some craft shops. I've also used ascorbic acid powder, or vitamin C, which works just as well.

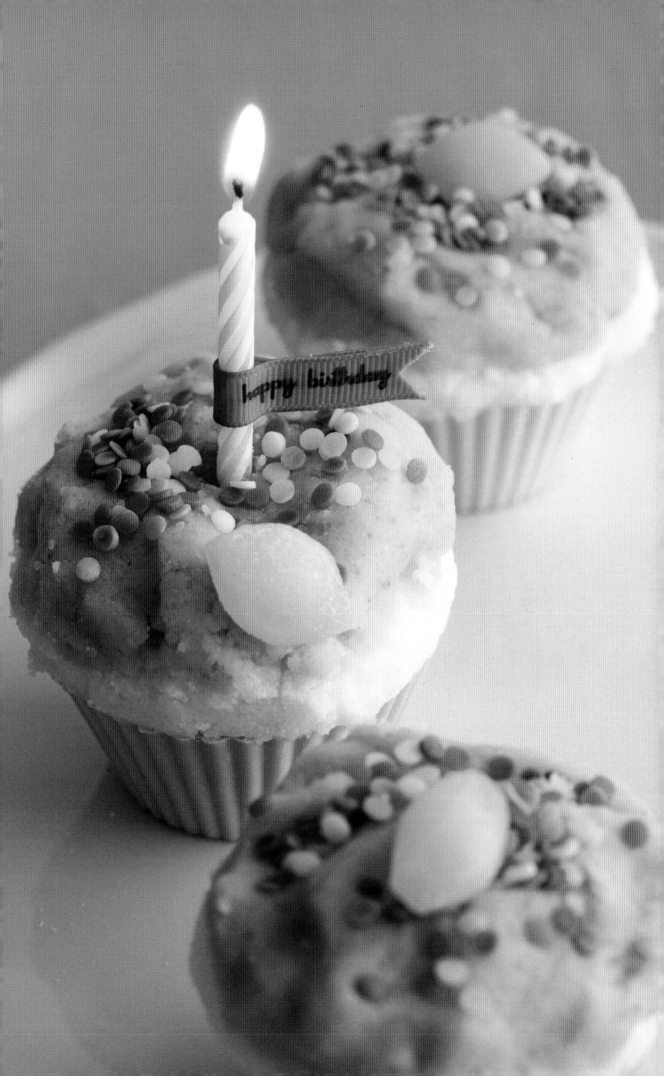

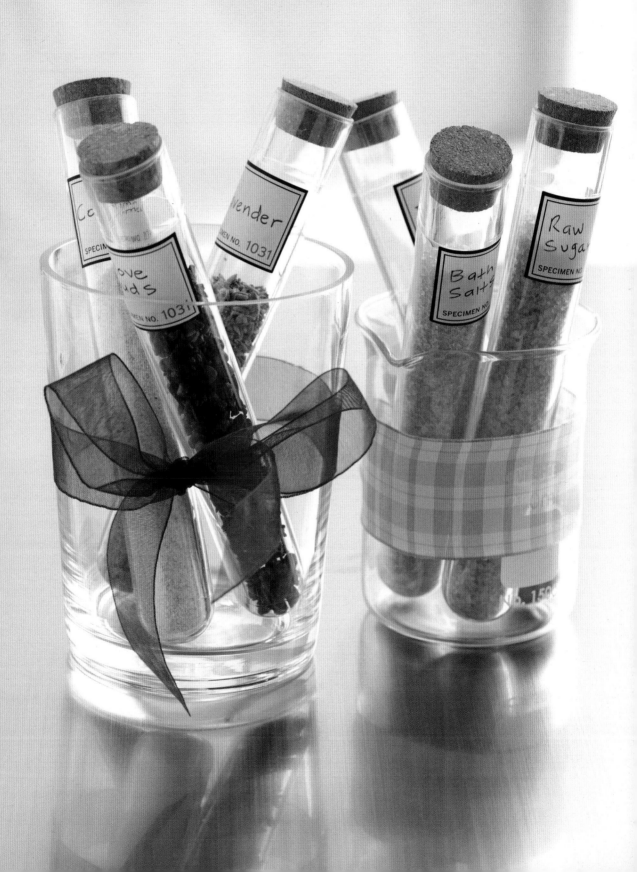

Cosmetics Chemistry Kit

I've always had a passion for science, so I'm especially fond of these cosmetics chemistry kits. It's sure to impress the recipient. You can find test tubes and science gear at some craft stores; if not, try looking in the yellow pages under chemical supplies. Another alternative is to use the tubes that beads or other small items come in, if you have them. Don't forget, reuse is the highest form of recycling!

6 glass or plastic test tubes

6 corks or stoppers

1 test tube rack, or a small cardboard box with holes cut out to hold the tubes upright

A few simple body care recipes typed up on recipe cards

Protective eye wear, rubber gloves, or a white cotton apron

Labels

6 (1-tablespoon) portions of different dry body care ingredients

Here are a few ideas for ingredients to include and the types of recipes they can be used in. In addition to providing a few typed-up recipes from this book, you should encourage the recipient to conduct some body care experiments of her own devising!

* Dry clays such as green or white: Mix it up with a bit of water or yogurt for a facial mask.

* Green tea and herbal teas such as chamomile: They can be made into herbal skin toners or baths.

* Bath salts: Add them to a warm bath.

* Raw sugar: Use it as a body scrub.

* Blue, white, or yellow cornmeal: Use it as a face or foot scrub.

* Ground sunflower seeds: Use them as a face scrub. Simply grind them in a food processor or coffee grinder. Try substituting them for the sugar in the Bye-Bye Blackheads Scrub, page 19.

* Dried citrus peels: Add them to baths, scrubs, or foot soaks.

* Clove buds: Chew them for a natural breath freshener or add to a mouthwash.

* Fennel seeds: Chew them for a natural breath freshener, or add them to baths.

* Dried flower petals, such as lavender, rose, or calendula: Add them to baths, masks, powders, and body scrubs.

Yield: 1 chemistry kit

Beauty Sleep Eye Pillow

These cute little pillows made from fabric scraps or old silk scarves are perfect for blocking out the world and letting you get some beauty sleep. They're filled with lavender for relaxation and flaxseed for bulk; you can find both at most natural food stores, and at well-stocked grocery stores. You'll need some basic sewing skills, or if you want to take the easy way out, just use fabric glue. When I have a lot on my mind or just need some time to myself, I play some low-key music and relax with my eye pillow.

2 rectangular pieces of cotton or silk fabric, measuring about 5 by 9 inches

1 cup whole flaxseeds

2 teaspoons dried lavender flowers or dried rosemary leaves

Stitch the two pieces of fabric together on three sides, leaving one short end open. If the fabric has an inside and outside, have the inside facing out before you stitch them together. Turn the pillow inside out, then combine the flaxseeds and lavender and fill the pillow with the mixture. Stitch the open end closed.

To use, lie down, place the pillow over your eyes, and relax. To soothe tired eyes, cool your eye pillow in the refrigerator before you use it.

Yield: 1 eye pillow

GREAT GIFT: SAT PREP

Create a relaxing gift for a friend before the SATs or finals week. Burn some relaxing tunes onto a blank CD, then put it in a gift basket, along with a homemade eye pillow, lavender essential oil, a calming face mask, and plenty of chocolate!

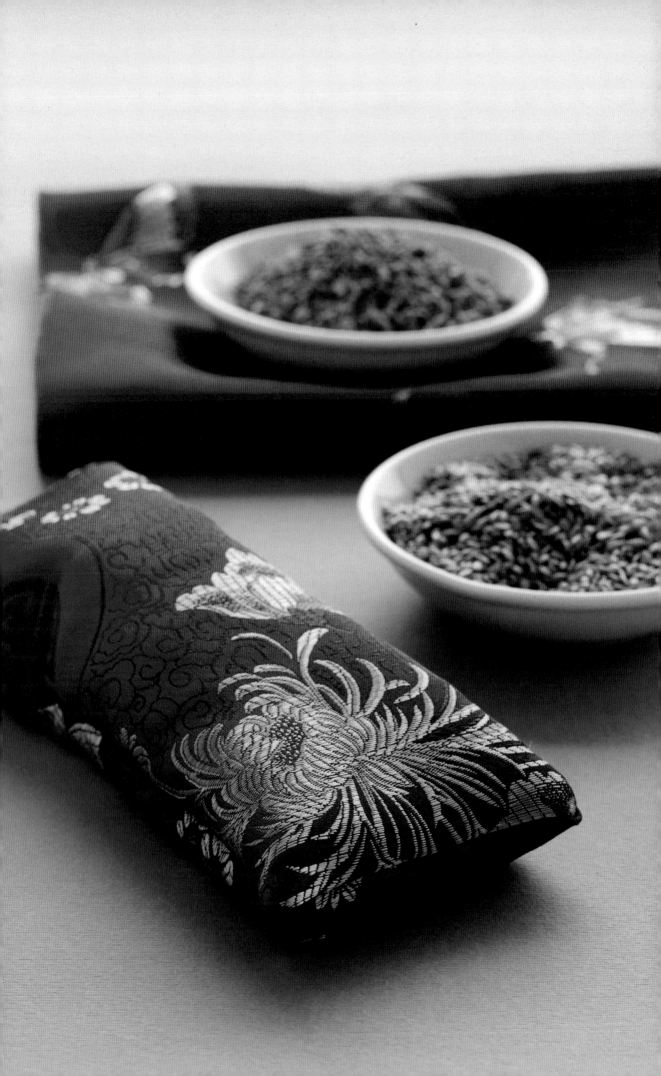

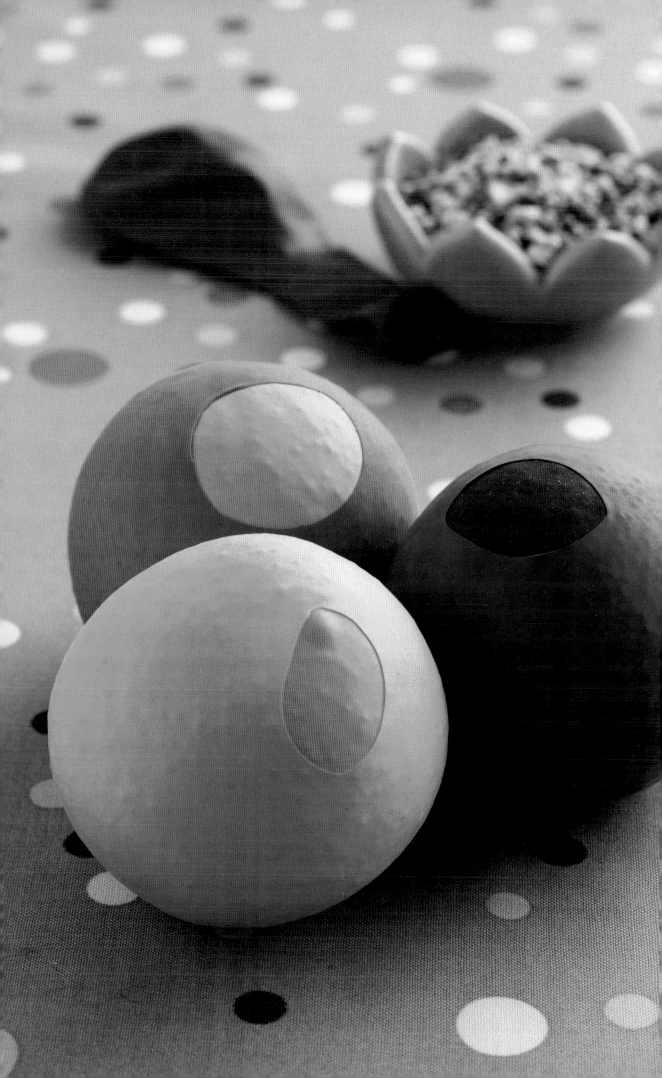

Stress Therapy Balls

I first saw these fun "juggling" balls, which make great fillers in gift baskets, at a market in Sydney, Australia. After buying a set and taking them apart, I discovered their secret—birdseed! I love to make these in bunches and keep a bowl of them in my dorm room. Squeezing them really does reduce stress, and they also help improve hand strength, making them a good gift for older relatives who suffer from arthritis. When I was in high school, a bunch of us made these for a local senior center. Oh, and you can also juggle with them if you're really talented!

¹/₂ cup fine birdseed (use
   something cheap, like millet)
1 small plastic sandwich bag
Tape
3 (9-inch-diameter) latex
   balloons

Pour the birdseed into the plastic bag, shape it into a small round package, and twist to close, then tape down the twisted end. Cut the long stem end off of the balloons. Stretch the first balloon around the plastic bag to cover it, then stretch the second balloon over the first, making sure to cover the cut edge. If you like, you can make small decorative slits or cuts in the last balloon. Stretch this over the second balloon. You now have a colorful ball to have fun with.

To use, gently squeeze the ball in your hand . . . or make a few and juggle with them.

Yield: 1 ball

ANOTHER GREAT GIFT IDEA

You can make your own cute and colorful beads from old magazines. Simply cut small triangles out of brightly colored pages and roll them up around a toothpick or bamboo skewer, starting with the wide end. Secure the pointy end with a bit of glue. Once the glue has dried, slide the beads off the toothpick and string them into a necklace or bracelet. For a hip, natural look, you can also include other beads, buttons, dried rose buds, small cinnamon sticks, star anise pods, and charms along with your magazine beads.

Popsicle Soaps

You scream, I scream, we all scream for . . . soap? I love creating molded soaps, especially these fun "popsicle" soaps; they make great summer gifts and party favors and couldn't be simpler to put together. I find popsicle molds at my local dollar store and wooden sticks at the craft store. Any colored glycerin soap will work in this recipe. For "multiflavored" popsicle soaps, layer different colors of melted soap into the molds, making sure each layer cools before adding the next one. To add a scent, get some flavored oils used for cooking and candy-making—these are usually less expensive than essential oils and come in fruity scents.

6 popsicle molds or
**   other plastic molds**
Coconut oil
2 to 3 bars of colored
**   glycerin soap**
Fruit-scented oil (optional)
6 wooden popsicle sticks

Grease the molds using a small amount of coconut oil. With a sharp knife, chop up the soap into small chunks, then put it in a microwave-safe container or a small saucepan. Microwave on low heat for 1 to 2 minutes, just until the soap is melted. If melting the soap on the stovetop, use low heat and cook, stirring occasionally, just until the soap is melted. Once the soap is melted, stir in the scented oil, then pour the soap into your molds. Cover the mold with plastic wrap or foil, then insert a wooden stick in the center of each "popsicle." Let the soap cool completely and set up, then remove the plastic wrap and unmold the soap. Wrap in a small plastic or cellophane bag, and tie a cute bow around the stick.

Yield: About 6 soaps (varies depending on mold size)

GREAT GIFT: MORE FUN SOAP IDEAS

Here are some other ways to have fun with molded soaps:

❋ Place small, heat-resistant plastic treasures such as bracelets, rings, or small rubber duckies in the molds before pouring in the melted soap.

❋ To make custom guest soaps, laminate digital photos and place them inside the molds before pouring in the melted soap.

❋ Sprinkle your molded soaps with glitter for sparkling results.

❋ For extra scrubbing power make "bath salt bars"; simply add rock salt to the melted soap just before pouring it into the molds.

❋ Slice thin circles from a loofah sponge with a bread knife, and put the slice in the molds before pouring in the melted soap.

❋ For a natural look, add dried citrus peels, flower petals, or herbs to the melted soap before pouring it into the molds.

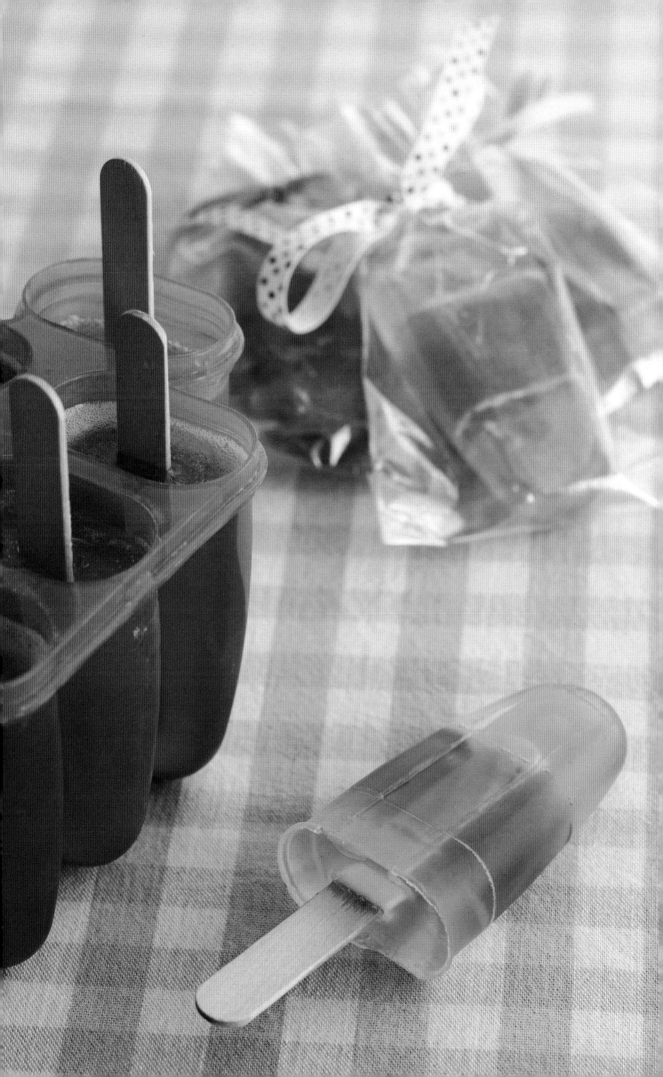

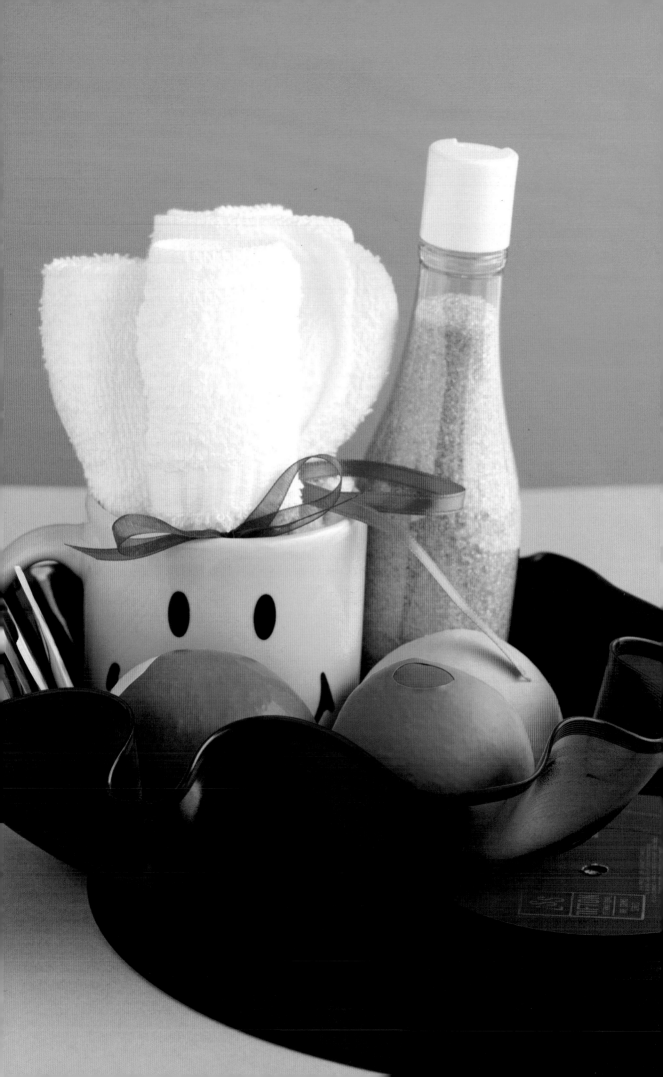

Rock 'n' Soap

These rock 'n' roll soaps make a great gift for the ultimate fan. Cut photos of a favorite rock group or artist out of a magazine. Then head to your local office supply store, where you can either have them laminated or purchase laminating sheets to do it yourself. Your soap molds can be anything from aluminum tart pans to plastic dishes—just make sure they're larger than your photos.

2 molds
Coconut oil
2 bars of clear glycerin soap
2 laminated photographs

Grease the molds using a small amount of coconut oil. With a sharp knife, chop up the soap into small chunks, then put it in a microwave-safe container or a small saucepan. Microwave on low heat for 1 to 2 minutes, just until the soap is melted. If melting the soap on the stovetop, use low heat and cook, stirring occasionally, just until the soap is melted. Place a laminated photo in the bottom of each mold, then pour the soap into each mold. Let the soap cool completely and set up, then unmold the soap.

Yield: About 2 soaps (depending on mold size)

Vinyl Record Bowl

I once found a bunch of old vinyl records at a used book sale and made them into cool bowls that were perfect containers for gifts like the Rock 'n' Soap, above. I still use one in my dorm room to hold some of my bath and beauty items. When melting records, it's a good idea to turn on the kitchen exhaust fan and open windows for ventilation.

Old vinyl record
2 (10-inch) ceramic
or glass bowls
Cookie sheet

Preheat the oven to 225°F. Place one of the bowls upside down on the cookie sheet, then put the record on top of it. Put the whole thing in the oven and leave it there for 5 minutes, until it begins to soften and melt. Remove it from the oven using the cookie sheet and quickly place the melted record inside the other bowl. You can now quickly shape it into whatever form you like. Once it cools completely, you'll have a record bowl. If you aren't happy with the shape, you can reheat the record bowl in the oven and try again, but don't sweat it too much. I think a free-form bowl is best.

Yield: 1 bowl

Easy Brown Paper Sack Basket

The easiest way to reuse a plain paper bag for gift giving is simply to decorate it. But if you want to go a step further, try making a sturdy basket with used paper grocery bags—or any kind of paper bag, as long as they're all the same size. The rolling process is fun, and you're sure to create a unique basket.

4 paper sacks, all the same size
A large-eyed sharp needle
Raffia or cotton string

Open up the first bag and gently roll the sides down until the top edge is about 1 inch from the bottom. Insert the next bag and roll its sides down until it meets the top edge of the first sack. Insert the third bag into the other two and roll its sides down until it meets the top edge of the second bag. You should now have a container or basket made up of three bags.

For the handle, take the fourth bag and cut the bottom out of it. Fold or roll down the sides until you have a complete circle. Slide this circle around the nested bags and position it in the center. Thread your needle with the string and stitch the handle in place, or even easier, just staple the handle on, then cover up the staples with a bow made of raffia or string.

You can decorate the basket using markers, paint, or stickers, or use a glue stick to attach shapes cut out of old newspapers, magazines, or junk mail.

Yield: 1 basket

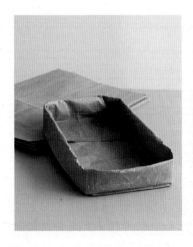 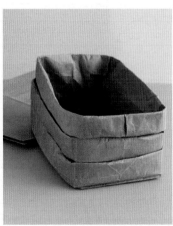 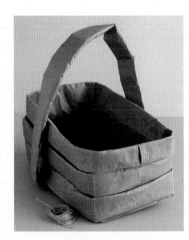

ECO TIP: Reduce waste when you're shopping by reusing old shopping bags or using your own cloth bag, and by buying products in bulk or with minimal packaging.

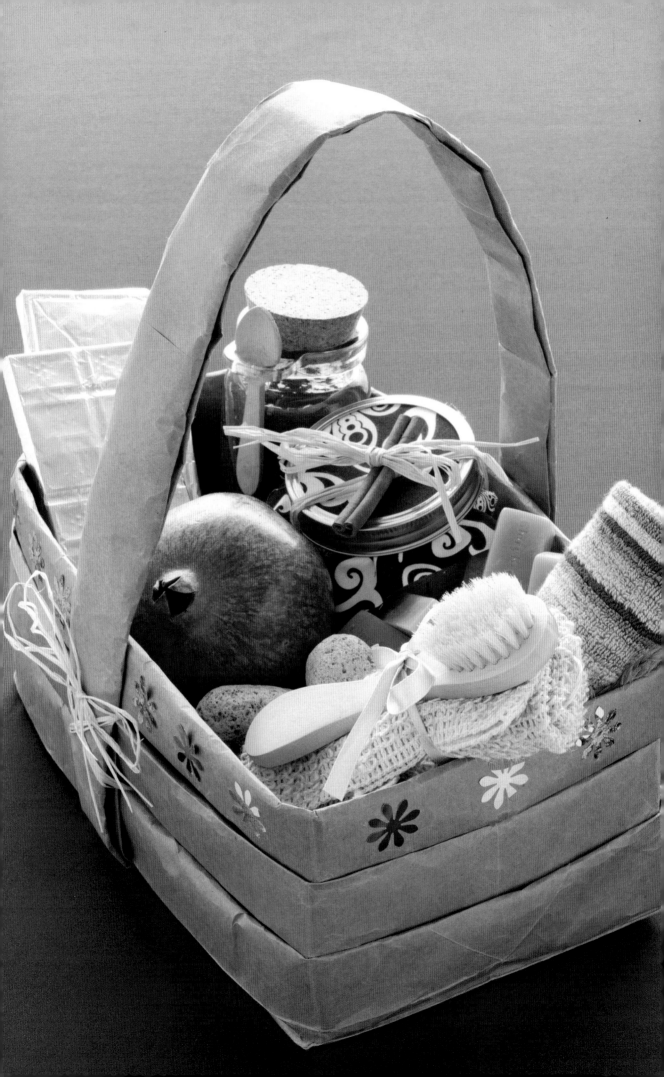

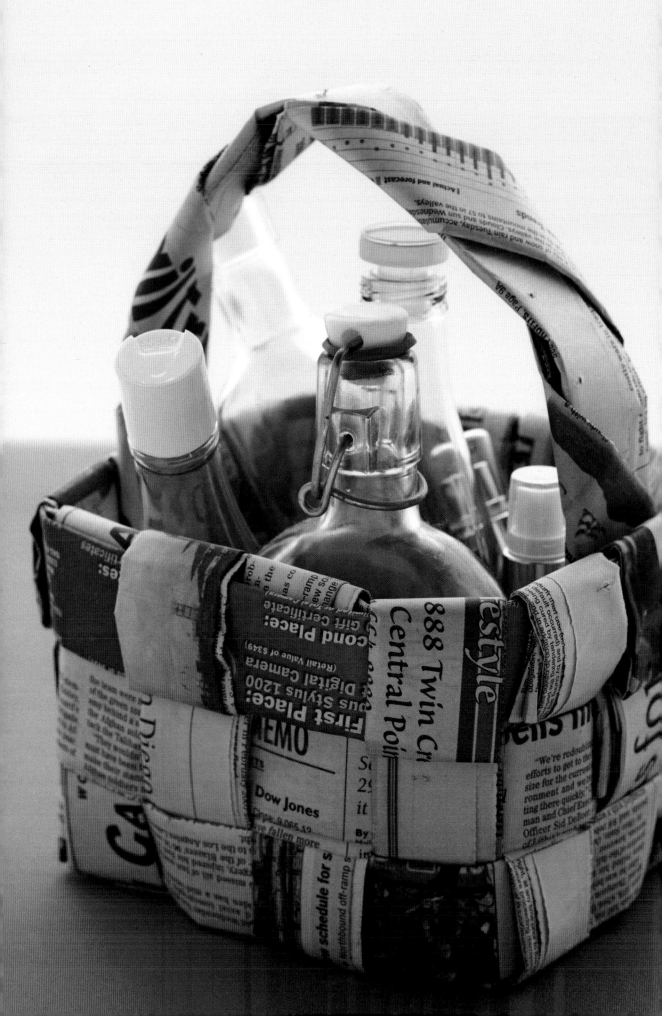

Woven Newspaper Basket

For fun, try using foreign newspapers, the comics pages from Sunday papers, or other colored newspapers to make this basket. A good source of different papers is the airport. I often pick up interesting papers left behind by fellow passengers when I travel and use them for decoupage projects and these baskets.

13 full sheets of newspaper
Tape
White glue
6 to 8 clothespins

Open up a sheet of newspaper, fold it in half widthwise, and continue folding until you have a long, 1 by 25-inch strip. Fold all 13 sheets this same way. Lay 3 strips side by side and weave 4 strips through them in the middle. Clip the 4 corners with clothespins to hold the strips in place; this is the base of your basket.

Take 1 strip and weave it over and under the strips all around the edges of the basket, securing it in place with the clothespins. Tape the two ends together; this is the start of the sides of your basket. Continue in the same way with 2 more strips.

For the basket top, place 1 strip around the top of all of the other strips and tuck all of the loose ends under or over it. Dab with some white glue to hold everything in place.

For the handle, take 2 strips and wrap one around the other and trim the ends. You may also want to secure the handle together with glue. Slide the handle into the sides of your basket, interweaving it, then tape or glue it in place.

Yield: 1 basket

COLLEGE SURVIVAL KIT

College is a new and scary time for most people. When I first went to college, I took this kit with me to help get me through the rough transition time. It will help anyone who feels a little homesick or just needs some TLC. Start with a Woven Newspaper Basket, or cover an old shoebox or empty cereal box with copies of favorite photos or cheerful pictures from magazines. The options for filling the kit are endless. I recommend a brightly colored washcloth, a cute toothbrush, herbal tea bags, energy bars, Scented Shower Gels (page 70), Cucumber After-Bath Splash (page 69), a Beauty Sleep Eye Pillow (page 136), and a mix CD with some great study songs.

Make a Difference!

I hope I've inspired you to create some of your own eco-friendly beauty products or add a new treatment such as a scrub or pedicure to your skin care regime. Earth-friendly, responsible beauty starts at home. Making your own products for yourself and your friends is not only a great way to have fun and get creative, it really will make our world a more beautiful place to live in.

Together we can make a difference. Small changes to something as basic as what we use to wash our face will add up if enough people start making eco-friendly choices. Making your own products and treatments at home will save you money, too, but perhaps more importantly, it also saves packaging, which in turn makes a difference in what's going into our land-fills and into our environment in general. In addition to developing good beauty hab-its, it's important to develop good habits to help beautify the earth, such as recycling and reducing waste. This can only benefit us in the future.

The recipes and ideas in this book offer a simple way to start making a difference. Being earth-friendly and looking your best really do go hand in hand, and you don't have to give up anything. In fact, in many ways, less is more when it comes to natural beauty. One of my mom's favorite state-ments is "We are all born with a natural beauty; it is how we choose to use it that makes us truly beautiful!" I couldn't agree more and would only add that each of us has only one body, and together we have only one world, so let's keep it beautiful.

EcoBeauty is better beauty for a bet-ter world. Each of us is amazing, and each of us can make a difference. Share your beauty!

Index